Mindfulness and Compassion in Integrative Supervision

Mindfulness and Compassion in Integrative Supervision presents an original integrative and transtheoretical approach to supervision that emphasises the importance of mindful awareness and compassion in supervision practice.

Psychotherapists are taught about the importance of compassion for their clients, while the role of bringing self-compassion toward themselves is often neglected. This book offers novel perspectives on mindful awareness, self-compassion, physiological synchrony, and emotional regulation in supervision. It presents various mindfulness- and compassion-oriented methods and interventions that are used within an attuned supervisory relationship. Through vignettes and transcripts of supervision sessions, the authors illustrate the power of mindful awareness and self-compassion to transform supervisees' dysregulated experience related to their psychotherapy work. The book embraces all main dimensions of human experience: Physiological, affective, relational, cognitive, behavioural, spiritual, and contextual.

The book will have an international appeal amongst supervisors from different supervision approaches and psychotherapists/counsellors who may find it useful for their practice, self-care, and the prevention of burnout.

Maša Žvelc, PhD, is an assistant professor of psychology at the University of Primorska. She is an international trainer and supervisor of integrative psychotherapy. She is the co-founder and director of the Institute for integrative psychotherapy and counselling, Ljubljana, where she leads the training in integrative psychotherapy and supervision. She is a co-author of the book *Integrative psychotherapy: A mindfulness- and compassion-oriented approach.*

Gregor Žvelc, PhD, is a full professor of clinical psychology at the University of Ljubljana. He is an international trainer and supervisor of integrative psychotherapy and transactional analysis. He is the co-founder of the Institute for integrative psychotherapy and counselling, Ljubljana, and the co-author of the book *Integrative psychotherapy: A mindfulness- and compassion-oriented approach.*

"This excellent book from two very experienced supervisors integrates the wisdom of mindfulness and compassion into the art and science of clinical supervision. It offers a deep dive into the many complexities of the therapeutic and the supervisory relationships. It highlights the importance of and ways of helping the supervisee be grounded in the body and settled in the mind, which facilitates openness to supervision and the long journey into developing mentalization and many other psychotherapy skills. I learnt much from this very accessible and richly informative volume and will be a repeat returner".

Paul Gilbert, *PhD, FBPsS, OBE, Professor of clinical psychology, University of Derby, President of the Compassionate Mind Foundation, Founder of Compassion Focused Therapy*

"Žvelc and Žvelc's masterful book on supervision invites the reader to embrace mindful awareness, interpersonal compassion, and self-compassion – essential process that facilitate a transformation of supervisee's possible emotional dysregulation and vicarious trauma into a calm therapeutic presence. While most mindfulness approaches focus on mindfulness and compassion as a technique to be learned by the client or therapist, the authors emphasize the importance of bringing mindfulness and compassion to the heart of the supervisory relationship, to the benefit of clients, supervisees, and supervisor".

Richard G. Erskine, *PhD, Institute for Integrative Psychotherapy; Professor of Psychology, Faculty of Health Sciences, Deusto, University, Bilbao, Spain*

"Themes of mindfulness and compassion have become increasingly prominent in the thinking of psychotherapists of widely varying orientations. Maša and Gregor Žvelc have brought the wisdom of innovative and integrative therapists to the application of these critical themes to the realm of supervision. In doing so, they have made a valuable contribution not only to our thinking about supervision but to our understanding of therapy as well".

Paul L. Wachtel, *Ph.D., Distinguished Professor, Doctoral Program in Clinical Psychology, City College of New York, Past President, Society for the Exploration of Psychotherapy Integration*

"Following on from their excellent book, Integrative psychotherapy: A mindfulness- and compassion-oriented approach, Maša and Gregor Žvelc bring us another application of their integrative approach, this time, to supervision. The authors offer the reader a lovely integration of theory with practice, with lots of vignettes. This is book which, while retaining its focus on supervision, brings and offers a breadth and depth of knowledge. Apart from their mindfulness and compassion for their supervisees, trainees, and colleagues – as well as the reader – authors also bring a generosity of spirit to these pages. I highly recommend this book".

Dr Keith Tudor, *Professor of Psychotherapy, Auckland University of Technology*

"This book is an essential resource for integrating mindfulness and compassion-oriented practice into supervision. Drs. Žvelc and Žvelc provide a thorough theoretical framework, along with tons of vignettes and exercises that supervisors can read today and use tomorrow. These lessons offer mental health professional innovative, yet practical ways to relate to themselves in times of difficulty and stress, a benefit they can pass along to their clients".

Susannah Coaston, *Ed.D., Associate Professor, Northern Kentucky University*

"In this groundbreaking and exciting book, Maša and Gregor Žvelc use the latest findings on physiological synchronization and memory reconsolidation to offer unique methods for developing mindfulness and compassion, first in the relationship between supervisor and supervisee and then between supervisee and client. Their transtheoretical, phenomenological, and experiential approach to supervision is intuitive and easily understood. The book is sure to become an excellent inspiration for supervisors and therapists of all contemporary schools of psychotherapy".

Jan Benda, *Ph.D., Charles University, Prague*

"This book by Maša and Gregor Žvelc is a superb addition to the supervision literature, a valuable resource for both beginning supervisees and those experienced in the field. It is an excellent follow-up to their book on Integrative psychotherapy, bringing a similar mindful, compassionate approach to supervision and emphasising the importance of here and now body awareness and autonomic regulation within the supervisory relationship. This is a treasure trove of a book, integrating theory and innovative ideas, practice and techniques".

Joanna Hewitt Evans, *Gestalt and Integrative Psychotherapist,*
Supervisor and Trainer in private practice, United Kingdom.
Secretary, European Association for Integrative Psychotherapy

"Žvelc and Žvelc have elegantly brought together a number of contemporary themes in psychotherapy practice and woven them into a research-based and coherent model for supervision. The book is rich with nuggets of wisdom that I am certain will inspire both new and experienced supervisors alike. By combining mindfulness with compassion-oriented principles, and current thinking on interoception and emotion regulation, Žvelc and Žvelc have developed a conceptual framework which will naturally lead to a deepening of reflection and increased capacity for here and now relational contact for both the supervisor and supervisee".

Mark Widdowson, *UKCP registered psychotherapist, senior lecturer in*
counselling and psychotherapy, University of Salford

Mindfulness and Compassion in Integrative Supervision

Maša Žvelc and Gregor Žvelc

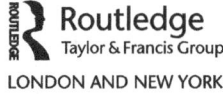
Routledge
Taylor & Francis Group

LONDON AND NEW YORK

Designed cover image: The Universal Essence by Amadej Žvelc, https://opensea.io/ArtTourNFTs

First published 2024
by Routledge
4 Park Square, Milton Park, Abingdon, Oxon OX14 4RN

and by Routledge
605 Third Avenue, New York, NY 10158

Routledge is an imprint of the Taylor & Francis Group, an informa business

British Library Cataloguing-in-Publication Data
A catalogue record for this book is available from the British Library

Library of Congress Cataloging-in-Publication Data
Names: Žvelc, Maša, 1973- author. | Žvelc, Gregor, 1974- author.
Title: Mindfulness and compassion in integrative supervision / Maša Žvelc and Gregor Žvelc.
Description: Abingdon, Oxon ; New York, NY : Routledge, 2024. | Includes bibliographical references and index. |
Identifiers: LCCN 2023010491 (print) | LCCN 2023010492 (ebook) | ISBN 9781032046556 (hardback) | ISBN 9781032046549 (paperback) | ISBN 9781003194118 (ebook)
Subjects: LCSH: Psychotherapists--Supervision of. | Mindfulness (Psychology) | Psychotherapists--Mental health.
Classification: LCC RC459 .Z94 2024 (print) | LCC RC459 (ebook) | DDC 616.89/14--dc23/eng/20230527
LC record available at https://lccn.loc.gov/2023010491
LC ebook record available at https://lccn.loc.gov/2023010492

ISBN: 978-1-032-04655-6 (hbk)
ISBN: 978-1-032-04654-9 (pbk)
ISBN: 978-1-003-19411-8 (ebk)

DOI: 10.4324/9781003194118

Typeset in Times New Roman
by MPS Limited, Dehradun

Contents

Figures, Tables, and Boxes

Figures

Tables

Boxes

Abbreviations

ANS   Autonomic Nervous System
MCIP   Mindfulness- and Compassion-Oriented Integrative Psychotherapy
MCIS   Mindfulness- and Compassion-Oriented Integrative Supervision
SPA   Scale of Physiological Arousal

Acknowledgements

We feel grateful to many people who have supported us and contributed to publishing this book.

We thank Routledge's editors, Grace McDonnell and Joanne Forshaw, and all team members who helped the book to see the light of day.

Special thanks to professor Clifton Edward Watkins for his kindness, support, and for writing the book's foreword.

We thank our supervisees, who agreed to publish the supervision vignettes from their supervision sessions. They enrich the book enormously.

We thank our colleague Robert Riley, who gave us crucial support for writing in English.

We thank our colleague Leticia Yebuah Slapnik for her help in designing figures.

We express sincere thanks to our supervision teachers and models: Ken Evans, Joanna Hewitt Evans, Richard G. Erskine, Geoff Hopping, Biljana van Rijn, Branko Franzl, and all others who raised us professionally. Your wisdom lives in us and is transmitted through this book.

We thank colleagues in our professional organisations who influenced our thinking and ideas: The International Integrative Psychotherapy Association (IIPA), the European Association for Integrative Psychotherapy (EAIP), and the Slovenian Association for Integrative Psychotherapy and Transactional Analysis (SINTA).

Gregor Žvelc acknowledges financial support from the Slovenian Research Agency (Research Core Funding No. P5-0110).

We thank our professional colleagues and trainees at the Institute for Integrative Psychotherapy and Counselling, Ljubljana, for your support and discussions that helped develop the ideas of this book.

We thank our sons, Lan and Amadej, for your patience and support during the writing of this book. We also thank Amadej for creating the image for the book cover.

We thank our parents for your unlimited support and for believing in us.

And last but not least, we thank each other for mutual support, fruitful discussions, and valuable corrections.

Maša Žvelc and Gregor Žvelc

Foreword

My blunt assessment: This is a FABULOUS, must-read supervision book! What awaits you, dear reader, is a uniquely innovative, consummately comprehensive, superbly structured, delightfully detailed, empirically founded, and grounded, case-abundant integrative approach to supervision. Stellar and masterful, this is indeed a masterwork – destined to be a richly revolutionary contribution to the clinical supervision literature.

Žvelc & Žvelc have crafted a roundly and soundly original perspective, trans-theoretical in nature, that gives loud and clear voice to some supremely significant supervision quintessentials – mindfulness, compassion, and self-compassion – whose inexorable interplay has been too long overlooked. Their wholistic vision of supervision, mindfulness- and compassion-oriented integrative supervision (MCIS), may well be the one and only supervision approach that is truly biopsychosocial in its very entirety. MCIS is an intersubjective vision that emphasises the interpersonal, cognitive, affective, physiological, behavioural, spiritual, and contextual dimensions of experience and their rumbling ramifications and, again, their inextricably intertwined interconnectedness, across the whole of the supervisory triad.

Furthermore, Žvelc & Žvelc present you with an approach that is compellingly *au courant* – as current as current could be, as in the know as you would ever hope to find, and as widely and deeply informed as could be imagined; as they make clear, MCIS integrates (a) elements from third-wave behavioural approaches that emphasise mindfulness and compassion and (b) research on memory reconsolidation, physiological synchrony, and polyvagal theory. Again, a revolutionary supervision approach informed by the most current thinking across several highly pertinent fields of study, seamlessly synthesised to maximal conceptual, practical, and empirical effect. A profoundly thought provoking read.

You subsequently will be treated to two robust MCIS book sections. The first section provides six chapters that powerfully present the core foundations and framework, the pillars of practice, for all that follows. Let me say that as a supervisor, I preeminently value knowing all of that upfront – the core values, principles, and frameworks that guide, and abide within, any supervisory approach. These first six chapters are exceptional, in my view, in explicating those very supervision matters, supervision's substrate, in exquisite detail – informing us, for example, with the greatest clarity about MCIS fundamental principles and core change processes, a framework for integrating mindfulness and compassion into supervision, a transformative supervision model, and an integrative model of supervision interventions. Žvelc & Žvelc, by means of those first six chapters, explicitly provide us with the ever so supremely solid ground upon which MCIS practice stands; they masterfully articulate and enunciate the "what" and "why" of their perspective (e.g. via rich explanations and illustrative case examples). Theirs is a most well-laid, elaborated foundation, *sans pariel* in its preparation for what comes next.

So, forever armed with and anchored in the "what" and "why" of MCIS practice (section one), we move on to its "how". The second section of the book again provides us with six chapters that powerfully present us with the very quintessentials of MCIS implementation and action – putting into practice the ("how to do it") values, principles, and frameworks of MCIS. That implementation and enactment are beautifully detailed via an abundance of rich intervention descriptions, intervention case examples, and intervention case transcriptions. As a supervisor, I also like to see by case example what exactly supervisors do during supervision, and I like to hear specifically what supervisors say to – their word-for-word interactions with – their supervisees in the very process of doing supervision. With this book, you are given a splendid and resplendent cornucopia of both, able to clearly and crisply see and hear what MCIS-informed supervisors do and say, how they put MCIS into practice and make it come alive in the supervisory situation across multiple supervision scenarios, across multiple supervision issues, and across multiple supervision contexts. What a wonderfully presented and ever informed and informing "let me specifically show you how" way to teach and learn. I must say that an immensely instructive read, an eminently exciting supervision treat, awaits you, dear reader.

May I say, too, in conclusion, a deeply heartfelt "thank you" to Drs. Žvelc and Žvelc, on their tremendously additive, tour de force contribution – a generative gift and promethean prize – to the psychotherapy supervision literature. Bravo, bravo, bravo!

C. Edward Watkins Jr. Ph.D.
Professor,
University of North Texas, and Trainer,
Institute of Psychotherapy,
Psychological Counselling and
Clinical Supervision

Introduction

Psychotherapists witness the darkest side of human experience. They face their clients' trauma and absorb emotional and physiological distress during psychotherapy sessions. Often, they cannot regulate these traumatic and dysregulated states and bring them to supervision. One of the vital aims of mindfulness- and compassion-oriented integrative supervision (MCIS) is to transform these dysregulated states into balanced states of mind with regulated emotions and physiology. This book shows how supervision can help transform the therapist's work-related anxiety, distress, and sorrow into dignity, compassion, love, and strength. This transformation of burdening countertransferential experiences can happen with the help of mindful awareness, compassion, and self-compassion. In MCIS, the supervisor promotes the supervisee's mindful awareness and self-compassion during supervision sessions, which helps to transform the supervisee's inner experience. MCIS pays particular attention to the supervisor's and supervisee's mindful body awareness and regulation of their physiological arousal. In MCIS, mindfulness and compassion are viewed as essential supervision processes used within an attuned supervisory relationship. The approach presented in this book is transtheoretical and can be used in different supervisory approaches.

The book's authors are integrative psychotherapists, supervisors, trainers, academic professors, and researchers. Maša Žvelc was trained in integrative relational supervision by Ken Evans and Joanna Hewitt Evans and certified by the International Integrative Psychotherapy Association (IIPA) and the European Association for Integrative Psychotherapy (EAIP). Gregor Žvelc was trained in integrative psychotherapy supervision by Richard G. Erskine and is certified within IIPA, EAIP, and as a teaching and supervising transactional analyst within the European Association for Transactional Analysis.

The authors of the book experienced the benefits of mindfulness and self-compassion in their lives and started to apply them in their psychotherapy and supervision practice. Over the years, they developed mindfulness- and compassion-oriented integrative psychotherapy (G. Žvelc & Žvelc, 2021) as an integration of relationally focused integrative psychotherapy with practice,

DOI: 10.4324/9781003194118-1

theory, and research in mindfulness and compassion. The development of MCIS is the next step. It aims to bring mindfulness and compassion to the heart of integrative supervision theory and practice.

This book presents the concepts and methods of MCIS and is divided into two parts. Part one includes the first six chapters and presents the main theoretical constructs of MCIS and the authors' own research findings on the supervision process. Theory and research are supported with examples and vignettes from research and supervision practice.

Chapter 1, "Introduction to mindfulness- and compassion-oriented integrative supervision", describes the development of mindfulness- and compassion-oriented integrative supervision (MCIS). The authors present MCIS's fundamental principles and core processes of change in supervision related to different dimensions of human experience: Interpersonal, cognitive, affective, physiological, behavioural, spiritual, and contextual. In MCIS, mindfulness and compassion are viewed as meta-processes of change that influence all other change processes.

Chapter 2, "Relating from the observing self: Mindfulness and compassion in supervision", provides the framework for integrating mindfulness and compassion in supervision. The authors describe three main models that help the supervisor understand and use mindfulness and compassion in supervision: The diamond model of the observing self, the triangle of relationship to inner experience, and the keyhole model of relational mindfulness and compassion. The keyhole model of relational mindfulness and compassion describes the main relational methods that invite the supervisee to relate fromthe observing self and bring mindful awareness and compassion into supervision and psychotherapy.

Chapter 3, "Mindfulness- and compassion-oriented transformative supervision model", presents the transformative supervision model, which explains how supervision, with the help of mindful awareness and self-compassion, transforms the supervisee's way of being and their dysfunctional relational schemas of being with the client. This positively affects the therapist's subsequent psychotherapy sessions.

In Chapter 4, "Emotional and physiological regulation as the fourth supervision function", the authors introduce the significance of emotional and physiological regulation in supervision based on supervision research, intersubjective physiology research, the concept of window of tolerance, and clinical practice. The authors discuss functional and dysfunctional physiological synchrony in supervision and how they relate to the effectiveness of psychotherapy and supervision practice. They elaborate on factors contributing to physiological dysregulated states in supervision and the significance of the physiological parallel process.

Chapter 5, "Supervisory alliance and supervisory alliance rupture repair", discusses contracting in supervision and factors contributing to a good supervisory bond. Examples of alliance ruptures and problematic supervision events are presented. The authors give directions for alliance rupture repair in supervision and illustrate how to apply them through a vignette from a supervisory session.

Chapter 6, "Methods and interventions in integrative supervision", introduces the integrative model of supervision interventions categorised into 1) interventions directed towards the supervisory relationship, 2) interventions focused on the supervisee, 3) Interventions directed towards case conceptualisation, 4) interventions focused on psychotherapeutic work, 5) working with a supervision group, 6) activity within the supervisor, and 7) interventions oriented to the psychotherapeutic and supervisory system. The authors illustrate each category with citations from their research, showing the practical use of the interventions.

Part two presents the methods and interventions that encourage mindful awareness, psychological regulation, and self-compassion in supervision. The authors illustrate these methods with numerous vignettes and verbatim transcripts from their supervision practice.

Chapter 7, "Mindfulness-oriented interventions in integrative supervision", presents exercises for mindful preparation for supervision and relational methods that promote core mindfulness processes in supervision: Present moment awareness, acceptance, and decentred perspective. The chapter presents various examples of mindfulness-oriented supervisory interventions, which are directed to different dimensions of the supervisee's experience: Physiological, affective, cognitive, behavioural, relational, and spiritual. The use of mindfulness-oriented interventions is also illustrated with the help of two vignettes.

Chapter 8, "Mindful processing in psychotherapy supervision", presents the mindful processing method used to transform and process the supervisee's countertransference experiences. The method involves structured moments of silence, where supervisees bring mindful awareness to their inner experience evoked by activation of the relational schema of being with the client. Supervisees alternate between mindful awareness of experience and sharing the experience with the supervisor. Mindful processing promotes the transformation of the supervisee's relational schemas of being with the client and positively impacts the subsequent psychotherapy session and the supervisee's well-being. Two vignettes with transcripts from supervision sessions illustrate mindful processing in supervision.

In Chapter 9, "Methods of emotional and physiological regulation in supervision", the authors introduce the Triple R model, which describes three main supervision tasks related to emotional and physiological regulation in supervision: 1. *Recognition* of emotional and physiological dysregulation, 2. *regulation* of physiology and emotions, and 3. *reflection* on the meaning of dysregulation. Two supervision vignettes illustrate this model and show the process of physiological regulation of the supervisee's hypoarousal and hyperarousal.

Chapter 10, "Compassion-focused interventions in integrative supervision", presents how to promote compassion and self-compassion within the supervision sessions. The authors present relational methods for promoting self-compassion that are used within the attuned supervisory relationship and several self-compassion exercises used for the self-care of both the supervisor and supervisee.

Chapter 11, "Self-compassion processing in supervision", introduces the self-compassion processing supervision method for transforming painful countertransference experiences. The authors present three fundamental phases of the self-compassion processing supervision method: 1) Leading the supervisee to mindful awareness of their painful experience, 2) promoting the supervisee's self-compassion, and 3) integration. The method is illustrated with two vignettes, one from the supervision of complex trauma therapy and the other from the supervision of couple therapy.

Chapter 12, "Self-care and prevention of burnout in mindfulness- and compassion-oriented supervision", presents how supervision, by promoting mindful awareness, self-compassion, and physiological regulation, encourages the supervisee's self-care and prevents burnout. The authors discuss the meaning of dysfunctional physiological synchrony, which contributes to the emotional distress of psychotherapists. They propose strategies for the prevention of burnout and self-care, linked to the acronym MANER: 1) MA – mindful awareness of body and physiological states, 2) NE – recognition of needs, and 3) R – regulation and building resources, and illustrate its use with three supervision vignettes.

It is our hope that this book will appeal to supervisors from different supervision approaches interested in promoting mindful awareness, compassion, and self-compassion in supervision. We also trust that it will benefit supervisors who are interested in using methods and interventions that focus on the physiological, emotional, and relational dimensions of human experience. In addition to supervisors, this book will also be of interest to psychotherapists and counsellors, who will find examples of their dilemmas and struggles illustrated in the supervision vignettes and who may thereby be encouraged to reflect on their psychotherapy work and supervision process.

Part 1

Theoretical foundations

Chapter 1

Introduction to mindfulness- and compassion-oriented integrative supervision

Mindfulness- and compassion-oriented integrative supervision (MCIS) is an approach that emphasises the importance of mindful awareness and compassion in supervision practice. It is a transtheoretical model of supervision that can be used within different supervision approaches. In MCIS, mindfulness and compassion are essential processes used within an attuned supervisory relationship to enhance supervisees' accepting awareness of their experience and compassion towards themselves and their clients. MCIS is an integrative, holistic approach encompassing different dimensions of human experience: Interpersonal, cognitive, affective, physiological, behavioural, spiritual, and contextual. It is a process-based supervision founded on processes of change that are the underlying mechanisms of effective supervision.

While supervision is often focused on a cognitive understanding of clients and the therapeutic relationship, MCIS emphasises optimising the supervisee's *way of being with the client*. Psychotherapists in the course of their professional practice often experience dysregulated emotional and physiological states, which may negatively impact their practice and personal life. In MCIS, we focus on supervisee's experiences related to their clients, enhance emotional and physiological regulation, and help them to transform their experience with the help of mindful awareness and self-compassion. This positively impacts the supervisee's subsequent psychotherapy sessions and is also vital for the supervisee's self-care and the prevention of burnout.

MCIS is a relational approach that gives importance to the supervisory alliance and supervision relationship. Supervision is viewed from an intersubjective perspective, where all members mutually influence one another. In addition to manifest phenomena, in MCIS, we are interested in latent, implicit, and unconscious processes, such as intersubjective physiology and parallel processes.

Development of mindfulness- and compassion-oriented integrative supervision

MCIS evolved from 1) mindfulness- and compassion-oriented integrative psychotherapy (G. Žvelc & Žvelc, 2021), 2) the integrative relational approach

DOI: 10.4324/9781003194118-3

to psychotherapy supervision (M. C. Gilbert & Evans, 2000), and 3) scientific research on supervision.

Mindfulness- and compassion-oriented integrative psychotherapy

MCIS is influenced by mindfulness- and compassion-oriented integrative psychotherapy (MCIP) that has its roots in relationally focused integrative psychotherapy developed by Richard G. Erskine and his colleagues (Erskine, 2015, 2020; Erskine & Moursund, 2011, 2022; Erskine et al., 1999, 2023). Relationally focused integrative psychotherapy is based on the theoretical integration of different psychotherapy approaches and the importance of common factors in psychotherapy, such as the therapeutic relationship.

We further integrated this approach with mindfulness- and compassion-oriented approaches, research, and practice. This resulted in the development of MCIP (G. Žvelc & Žvelc, 2021). MCIP integrates acceptance and commitment therapy (S. C. Hayes et al., 2012) and elements from other third-wave behavioural approaches that emphasise the importance of mindfulness and compassion. It integrates research on memory reconsolidation (Ecker, 2015, 2018; Ecker et al., 2012; Lane et al., 2015), physiological synchrony (Kleinbub et al., 2020; Palumbo et al., 2017), and elements from the poly-vagal theory (Porges, 2011, 2017).

In MCIP, the "qualities of mindfulness and compassion are at the heart of the therapeutic relationship" (G. Žvelc & Žvelc, 2021, xv). Mindfulness and compassion are understood as meta-processes of change that are enhanced within an attuned therapeutic relationship. MCIP differs from some other third-wave approaches as it is not primarily focused on teaching clients mindfulness and compassion techniques. Although the therapist may teach clients some mindfulness techniques, the primary goal is to bring mindfulness and compassion into the therapeutic relationship. In this way, it prioritises the mindful and compassionate presence of the therapist and relational methods that invite the client to bring mindfulness and compassion towards their inner experience or parts of self.

Mindfulness- and compassion-oriented supervision was influenced by the theories and ideas that were developed within MCIP. The practice of MCIS shares with its psychotherapy cousin the central premise that mindfulness and compassion processes are used relationally and are brought into the super-visory relationship. We invite the supervisee to bring mindfulness and compassion towards their inner experience while discussing their client. This leads to fresh insights, physiological regulation, and processing of the counter-transference experiences. The mindful and compassionate presence of the supervisor is also essential in this approach, as it promotes these qualities in the supervisee.

In MCIS, we use theoretical models of mindfulness and compassion developed within MCIP: The diamond model of the observing self, the triangle of relationship to internal experience, and the keyhole model of relational mindfulness and compassion (see Chapter 2). We also pay special attention to the process of physiological synchrony and provide emotional and physiological regulation during supervision (see Chapters 4 and 9).

The integrative relational approach to psychotherapy supervision

MCIS is influenced by the integrative relational approach to psychotherapy supervision developed by Ken Evans and Maria Gilbert (M. C. Gilbert & Evans, 2000). This approach to psychotherapy supervision gives primacy to the psychotherapeutic and the supervisory relationship (M. C. Gilbert & Evans, 2000). Its philosophical roots are in phenomenology, constructivism, and field theory. It is based on object relations theory, attachment theory, and the intersubjective perspective. The intersubjective perspective focuses on the interactional field created by two or more people (Stolorow, 1994). It emphasises that personal reality is always co-determined by the context. The integrative relational approach uses an intersubjective perspective on unconsciousness processes, such as transference, countertransference, and the parallel process (Taylor et al., 2006). It uses a meta-system perspective, the concept of the I-It and I-Thou relationship (Buber, 1999), and Sullivan's concept of the participant-observer (M. C. Gilbert & Evans, 2000). This approach to supervision also focuses on dealing with shame, raising multicultural perspective awareness, and skills for anti-oppressive practice. MCIS is based on these same core principles of integrative relational supervision (M. C. Gilbert & Evans, 2000).

Research on supervision

MCIS is based on our research on the supervision process (M. Žvelc, 2015, 2017; M. Žvelc & Žvelc, 2021) and other supervision research regarding helpful and hindering processes in supervision, the supervisory alliance, and research into mindfulness and compassion for mental health professionals. Throughout the book, we provide references to numerous studies that influenced the core ideas and concepts of MCIS.

In her doctoral dissertation, Maša Žvelc researched facilitating and hindering factors in supervision (M. Žvelc, 2017). Her fundamental research question was related to the exploration of what is effective in supervision and what hinders the supervision process from the perspective of supervisees and their supervisors. Pairs of supervisees (N = 50) and their supervisors (N = 12) from different psychotherapy approaches completed a questionnaire about the helpful aspects of the supervision session (M. Žvelc, 2015, 2017). Participants chose and described the most significant events in the supervision session, the hindering events in the supervision session, and any occurrence of non-disclosure. Supervisors were also asked which methods and interventions in their opinion led to the significant events. A total of 90 completed questionnaires were included in the final analyses. Afterwards, semi-structured interviews were conducted with ten supervisees who experienced supervision either as very helpful or very hindering. Based on the qualitative analyses of the questionnaires and transcripts from interviews, M. Žvelc (2017) developed several models of supervision that have influenced the theory of MCIS. In our book, we present the following models that were influenced by her research: 1) The integrative model of processes of change (presented later in this chapter), 2) the integrative model of the supervisor's interventions (see Chapter 6), and 3) the model of resolution of alliance ruptures in supervision (see Chapter 5).

Fundamental principles of mindfulness- and compassion-oriented integrative supervision (MCIS)

In the following sections, we explain the fundamental principles of MCIS that underpin its theory and methods.

Mindful awareness and compassion as core processes in supervision

In MCIS, mindful awareness and compassion are viewed as core processes of change. The essential task of the supervisor is to help the supervisee to bring mindful awareness to their experience. By accepting awareness of thoughts, fantasies, emotions, and physiological sensations, supervisees gain new insights regarding themselves and their relationship with the client. Mindfulness and compassion processes in supervision also bring physiological and emotional regulation to the supervisee and have transformative power. Mindful awareness and self-compassion help transform the supervisee's emotional and bodily felt experience of the client. This helps the supervisee to be more present, compassionate, and have greater ability for mentalisation.

As supervisees are often highly critical of themselves, the process of self-compassion helps the supervisee to experience kindness and love towards themselves. This helps them to develop greater inner acceptance and compassion towards their client. Psychotherapeutic work is often emotionally demanding and painful, which may lead to empathic distress and burnout. With the help of mindful awareness and compassion in supervision, we help supervisees to ease their burden of self-doubt, self-criticism, and emotional distress connected to their work. Mindful awareness and self-compassion are essential for self-care and the prevention of burnout.

Relational approach and intersubjectivity

MCIS is rooted in the relational paradigm, which is based on the fundamental principle that people are interconnected and influence each other. We look at the supervision process as an intersubjective field (Stolorow, 1994), where all members mutually co-create the supervisory relationship. We also pay attention to a larger field, the intersubjective field, that includes the client, therapist, and supervisor. There is a mutual influence between the client–therapist and supervisee–supervisor dyads. In MCIS, we pay attention to the parallel process between these dyads and, through transformative changes in the supervisor–supervisee dyad, affect changes in the client–therapist matrix.

In addition to manifest phenomena, we are also interested in latent, implicit, and unconscious processes. We apply the concept of *intersubjective physiology* (G. Žvelc & Žvelc, 2021) to supervision. The concept of intersubjective physiology describes how humans affect each other automatically on a physiological level (G. Žvelc & Žvelc, 2021). People tend to synchronise their heartbeat, heart rate variability, volume and frequency of breathing, skin conductivity, levels of hormones, etc. (Palumbo et al., 2017). We apply these findings to supervision theory and practice. In MCIS, we aim to understand the interplay of physiological synchrony between supervisor and supervisee and its connectedness to the primary client–therapist relationship. The supervisor in MCIS takes the role of the "leader", who leads the dysregulated supervisory field towards regulation. With the help of mindfulness, compassion, and physiological regulation, we aim towards a regulated supervisory field that can influence the primary client–therapist system.

Holism and the importance of all dimensions of human experience

MCIS is an integrative form of supervision that is holistic and emphasises all dimensions of human experience: Physiological, affective, cognitive, behavioural, relational, spiritual, and contextual. It is based on processes of change related to all dimensions of human experience. Later in this chapter, we describe the integrative model of processes of change that describe the core change processes of effective supervision.

Significance of emotional and physiological regulation in supervision

We view emotional and physiological regulation as the essential function of supervision. Therapists often synchronise with their clients' dysregulated physiology and bring these dysregulated states into supervision. The supervisor's task is to help supervisees recognise emotional and physiological dysregulation, help them regulate themselves, and reflect on the meaning of it. In this way, the supervisee's emotions and physiology are brought back into the window of tolerance (D. J. Siegel, 1999, 2012). This then enables them to tolerate their emotions, to be open to learning, and to be able to think flexibly. Emotional and physiological regulation in supervision helps supervisees to be mindfully present and in contact with themselves and others. The supervisees are then able to bring these states of optimal arousal, safeness, and presence to the following therapy sessions. Emotional and physiological regulation posi-tively affects supervisees' work with clients and their own well-being.

The transformative nature of supervision

MCIS is based on the transformative supervision model (see Chapter 3). This proposes that the important task of supervision is to facilitate a change in the supervisee's way of being with their client and, consequently, the transforma-tion of their dysfunctional relational schemas of being with the client through the memory reconsolidation process (Ecker et al., 2012; Lane et al., 2015). In MCIS, we see supervision as a transformative process that can transform the supervisee's way of being related to their experience with the client. Processes of mindful awareness, compassion, and emotional and physiological regulation help regulate and transform their bodily felt client experience. Transformation of the supervisee's experience of the client may change their dysfunctional relational schemas of being with the client and positively impact subsequent psychotherapy sessions. By transforming the supervisee's way of being, the supervisee enters the next psychotherapy session with changed physiology and emotional experience, which promotes mindful presence, and compassion towards the client and enhances their ability for mentalisation.

The experiential and phenomenological approach to supervision

MCIS is an experiential and phenomenological approach to supervision that respects and values supervisors' and supervisees' phenomenological experiences.

In MCIS, we encourage mindful awareness of the supervisee's experience occurring here-and-now in supervision rather than only discussing their cognitive view of the client and psychotherapy relationship. In addition to the verbally based consultation process, MCIS emphasises the bottom-up pro-cess, where meanings and insights emerge through the supervisee's mindful awareness of bodily felt experience.

MCIS is a phenomenological approach in which we value supervisees' subjective here-and-now experiences in supervision as important communi-cation regarding themselves and their relationship with the client. We de-centre from our theories and ideas to make space for the supervisee's experience. At the same time, we stay present and in contact with ourselves, starting with mindful awareness of our bodies. We may then share our ex-periences and ideas as subjective "truths" rather than objective realities.

Importance of relationships and supervisory alliance

As a relational form of supervision, MCIS assumes that the need for human relationships is a primary human motivation. We emphasise the importance of a good supervisory alliance and actively work on resolving ruptures in the alliance. MCIS is an experiential supervision approach where supervisees are invited to mindful awareness and compassion towards themselves and others. Supervisees can mindfully observe and share their inner experience only in the presence of a supervisor with whom they feel secure. Security in the supervisory relationship is a prerequisite for all other interventions used in MCIS.

Processes of change in MCIS

A number of process-based psychotherapies have emerged, which present a new paradigm in clinical science (S. C. Hayes & Hofmann, 2018; Hofmann & Hayes, 2019). Instead of focusing on the treatment of different clinical disorders, this paradigm focuses on empirically validated transdiagnostic processes of change (Hofmann & Hayes, 2019). Processes of change are core underlying mechanisms of change that can be enhanced by different methods and interventions. In MCIP, we developed the integrative model of processes of change that describes processes of change related to the main dimensions of human experience (G. Žvelc & Žvelc, 2021). In line with this model, we have formulated the core change processes that are central to our supervision approach.

MCIS is a process-based supervision model founded on evidence-based processes of change that facilitate supervision effectiveness. Processes of change in supervision are core mechanisms of supervision that lead to the attainment of specific supervision goals. The model of processes of change in integrative supervision (see Table 1.1) offers an integrative conceptualisation of supervision processes that encompasses all dimensions of human experience. The model was inspired by the integrative model of processes of change in integrative psychotherapy (G. Žvelc & Žvelc, 2021). The change processes described in the model are based on our research in supervision (M. Žvelc, 2015, 2017) and findings of other contemporary supervision studies and authors that describe factors of effective supervision (Crunk & Barden, 2017; Lampropoulos, 2003; Watkins, 2017a, 2018b).

Based on the qualitative analysis of her research findings, M. Žvelc (2017) described the following facilitative factors in supervision: 1) Good supervisory alliance, 2) openness, presence, and attunement of the supervisor, 3) the supervisor's effective interventions, 4) the supervisee's insight, reflection, and mentalisation, 5) changes in the supervisee's experience, 5) practice of skills by the supervisee, and 6) emotional regulation. These facilitative factors can be described as meta-theoretical common supervision factors, as they were found across different theoretical supervision backgrounds and psychotherapeutic approaches. The findings of M. Žvelc (2017) are congruent with Watkins's (2017a, 2018b) and Lampropoulos's (2003) view of common supervision factors. For example, Watkins (2018b) emphasises three fundamental commonalities of the supervisor's contribution to the supervision goals: The supervisor's person and personhood, the supervisory relationship, and the supervisor's skills and interventions.

Table 1.1 The integrative model of processes of change in integrative supervision

META-PROCESSES OF CHANGE	
MINDFULNESS AND COMPASSION	Present moment awareness Decentred perspective Acceptance Self-compassion and compassion
DIMENSION OF HUMAN EXPERIENCE	**PROCESSES OF CHANGE**
INTERPERSONAL	Attunement Maintaining and repairing supervisory alliance
COGNITIVE	Understanding the client and the therapeutic process Self-reflection and mentalisation
AFFECTIVE	Awareness and acceptance of emotions Emotional regulation
PHYSIOLOGICAL	Interoception Physiological regulation
BEHAVIOURAL	Practising new skills/deliberate practice
SPIRITUAL	Contact with values and meaning related to psychotherapy practice Observing/transcendent self
CONTEXTUAL	Understanding contextual issues Reflection on ethics and standards of professional practice

Based on research findings of common facilitative factors of supervision and factors specific to the MCIS approach, we formulated the core change processes in integrative supervision as related to the main dimension of human experience. Table 1.1 presents the processes of change that are relevant for each of the main dimensions of human experience: Interpersonal, cognitive, affective, physiological, behavioural, spiritual, and contextual. Processes of mindfulness and compassion are presented as meta-processes of change that are related to all other dimensions.

We propose that these processes of change are meta-theoretical and are significant in different supervision approaches. However, supervision approaches differ in the attention given to a particular change process. In integrative supervision, we are flexible and work with all change processes as needed. The model includes both common factors of supervision and specific factors of change. In MCIS, mindfulness and compassion processes are specific to our approach and are seen as meta-processes of change that influence all other dimensions.

In integrative supervision, we assess which change process would be most beneficial to enhance at a particular moment based on the supervision goals and needs of the supervisees. The different methods and interventions, as described in Chapter 6, facilitate processes of change in supervision.

In MCIS, we place particular importance on the processes of **mindfulness and compassion**: *Present moment awareness, acceptance, decentred perspective, self-compassion, and compassion.* An increasing body of evidence shows that these processes significantly benefit clients' and practitioners' mental health. In MCIS, we invite the supervisee to bring mindful awareness to their experience and enhance compassion for themselves and their clients. Mindfulness and compassion are meta-processes of change that influence other change processes related to the main dimensions of human experience (G. Žvelc & Žvelc, 2021). Mindfulness, for example, enhances awareness and acceptance of emotions (Lindsay & Creswell, 2019; Teper & Inzlicht, 2013), emotional regulation (Farb et al., 2012; A. M. Hayes & Feldman, 2004; Hölzel et al., 2011; Teper & Inzlicht, 2013) and interoception (Farb et al., 2015). Self-compassion is also related to emotional regulation (Bates et al., 2021; Finlay-Jones, 2017; Inwood & Ferrari, 2018; Scoglio et al., 2015). We describe mindfulness and compassion processes in detail in Chapter 2.

The processes related to the **interpersonal dimension** are 1) attunement and 2) maintaining and repairing the supervisory alliance. In our research on supervision, the supervisor's openness, presence, and attunement were found to be important facilitative factors (M. Žvelc, 2017). Attunement is empathic sensing of another person's emotions, needs, and sensations and responding with a resonating response (Erskine & Trautmann, 1996). Attunement provides a sense of safety in supervision and a sense of being deeply understood. The supervisory alliance is another facilitative factor we found in our research and is the main common factor in supervision (Watkins, 2017a). The supervisory alliance consists of three mutually connected components: Agreement on supervision goals, agreement on supervision tasks, and the bond between the supervisor and the supervisee (Bordin, 1983). Ruptures in the supervisory alliance can impact the quality of supervision (Vîşcu & Watkins, 2021; M. Žvelc, 2017). Working with ruptures in the supervisory alliance is therefore necessary for repairing and maintaining a good supervisory alliance. Chapter 5 is focused on this essential process in supervision.

The processes related to the **cognitive dimension** are 1) understanding the client and the therapeutic process and 2) self-reflection and mentalisation. *Understanding the client and the therapeutic process* is fundamental to supervision and is used in most supervision approaches. It may involve case conceptualisation, treatment planning, and selection of methods and interventions. The second change process is *self-reflection and mentalisation*, which could be described as the meta-cognitive common factor in supervision (M. Žvelc, 2017). Bateman and Fonagy (2016) describe mentalisation as the ability to understand the mental states that underlie our own or other people's behaviour. One of the primary roles of the supervisor is to facilitate the supervisee's self-reflection and mentalisation regarding their relationship with their client and/or supervisor. It is an internal process where the supervisee distances, observes, and critically evaluates their own experience and reactions concerning the client's or supervisor's mental states (M. Žvelc, 2017).

The core change processes related to the **affective dimension** are 1) awareness and acceptance of emotions and 2) emotional regulation. *Awareness and acceptance of emotions* relate to full experiential contact with emotions that occur here and now in the supervision process. This factor is specific to MCIS and other experiential supervision approaches. Supervisees are often unaware of their emotional experience or try to avoid it, which negatively affects their work with their client and their mental health. With awareness and acceptance of emotions in supervision, we help supervisees regulate and process their emotions related to their work with clients. Awareness and acceptance of emotions are closely related to *emotional regulation*, as they help regulate emotions. However, emotional regulation also involves other processes, such as mentalisation, which helps understand emotions and put emotional experiences into words (symbolisation). Supervisees often come to supervision with dysregulated emotions, manifesting in either numbing or being overwhelmed with emotions. Dysregulated emotion impairs their ability for self-reflection and their ability for appropriate interventions in psychotherapy. They are also one of the supervisees' primary sources of burnout and somatic complaints. One of the important goals of supervision is therefore emotional regulation. In MCIS, the supervisor helps supervisees to regulate and reach the optimal zone of arousal – the window of tolerance (D. J. Siegel, 1999). This is related to a moderate level of emotional arousal, neither too high to be overwhelming nor too low to be distanced from emotions (Lane et al., 2015). This also enables optimal mental functioning and mentalisation.

The main processes related to the **physiological dimension** are 1) interoception and 2) physiological regulation. These two processes are specific to our mindfulness- and compassion-oriented approach. In MCIS, we place particular importance on bodily felt experience. We regularly invite supervisees to become mindfully aware of their bodily sensations in the present moment. Through accepting awareness of bodily sensations, supervisees come into contact with subsymbolic experience that underlies emotions, cognitions, and verbal narratives. Contact with bodily sensations enhances *interoception*, a "process of receiving, accessing, and appraising internal bodily signals" (Farb et al., 2015, p. 1). Awareness of bodily signals gives us essential information regarding emotions and the meaning of the current situation. By awareness of body sensations, supervisees gain new insights and meanings regarding their experience of their clients, which is often more salient than if they were only to cognitively discuss their clients. Interoception also promotes physiological and emotional regulation (Price & Hooven, 2018).

In this way, it is connected to the second primary process related to the physiological dimension – physiological regulation.

Supervisees' autonomous nervous systems are often dysregulated, which shows either in hyperarousal or hypoarousal. Physiological dysregulation negatively impacts all mental processes of the supervisee and can negatively impact their psychotherapy practice and supervision process. One of the main tasks of MCIS is promoting *physiological regulation*. The aim of physiological regulation in supervision is that the supervisee will enter the next psychotherapy session with regulated physiology and will be able to stay within the window of tolerance. Through self-regulation in supervision, supervisees learn this vital skill and how to use it within psychotherapy sessions with themselves and their clients. Chapters 4 and 9 of this book relate to this important supervision process.

Practising new skills is a change process related to the **behavioural dimension**. This change process is a common factor in supervision and was also found in our research to be a significant facilitative factor (M. Žvelc, 2017). Supervisees can practise new skills related to learning new interventions and methods or skills related to internal activity, such as physiological regulation or mindful awareness. This may involve the deliberate practice of specific skills that are essential in psychotherapy. Deliberate practice is an effective way to learn psychotherapy (Rousmaniere, 2017). In MCIS, we may use audio or videotapes of psychotherapy sessions and stop them at significant moments of the psychotherapy process. Supervisees are then invited to practice new ways of responding to the client. Such practice may involve the supervisee's inner activity, such as mindful awareness of emotions, or concrete interventions that are put into words. Practising new skills may also happen through role play of the client and the therapist, where the supervisor and supervisee play either role. Supervisees can, by modelling, learn new skills as they experience the supervisor in clinical action from the eyes of the client. After being in the role of the client, they may change their roles and the supervisee practises the role of the therapist.

The main processes related to the **spiritual dimension** in supervision are 1) contact with values and meaning connected to psychotherapy practice and 2) contact with the observing/transcendent self. Values guide our lives and give our life meaning and purpose (Luoma et al., 2007). Psychotherapists can lose a sense of meaning and purpose in their work because of client overload or painful experiences with their clients. They may become unmotivated and practice mechanically without passion and heart. In MCIS, we help supervisees regain contact with their meaning and purpose. Awareness and contact with inner values often impact the supervisee's motivation and may help them endure difficult times as they find meaning and a higher purpose in their work.

The observing/transcendent self is another important process in our approach that helps supervisees observe themselves and their clients from a broader perspective – the context of their experience. The observing/transcendent self is our essential self and could be described as *self-as-awareness*

(G. Žvelc & Žvelc, 2021). It is a perspective through which we observe our experiences and has transcendent properties (Deikman, 1982; S. C. Hayes et al., 2012; G. Žvelc & Žvelc, 2021). It is an aspect of ourselves that "metaphorically cannot be looked at but instead must be looked from" (Hayes et al., 2012, p. 85). The observing/transcendent self is the source of mindful awareness and compassion and has positive qualities related to transcendence, interconnection, stability, and containment (G. Žvelc & Žvelc, 2021). The process of the observing self helps supervisees experience themselves and their clients from a secure perspective; it helps them to contain and regulate emotions and feel compassion for themselves and their clients. The experience of self-compassion and compassion for others is often related to experiences of interconnection and love that are often felt as profound spiritual experiences.

Issues arising in supervision can also be related to the **contextual dimension**. The main processes related to this dimension are as follows: a) Understanding contextual issues and b) reflection on ethics and standards of professional practice.

Psychotherapists and supervisors work within larger systems that may influence their clinical practice, such as state laws, culture, family, and work environment. A significant supervision process connected to the understanding of contextual issues is addressing multicultural challenges and raising multicultural awareness (M. C. Gilbert & Evans, 2000; Ladany et al., 2005). The supervisor, the supervisee, and the client come from specific sociocultural groups (gender, sexual orientation, ethnicity, race, socioeconomic status, disability, religion, and family structure) (Ladany et al., 2005). It is important to consider the interplay between the different multicultural positions they may be in and how this can influence supervision and psychotherapy work. In recent years, other contextual factors have influenced psychotherapy and supervision practice, such as issues related to the covid pandemic, the war in Ukraine, and economic issues such as inflation.

Understanding the context of the psychotherapists' work environment and their relationships with other professionals and professional organisations are also important topics in supervision. Psychotherapists cooperate with other professionals, such as general practitioners, psychiatrists, nurses, or lawyers. Their work is also undertaken within professional psychotherapy organisations or chambers. Supervisees' issues related to their personal life and family environment (for instance, divorce, death of family members, or illness) may significantly influence the supervisee's psychotherapy practice and are issues that may emerge in the supervision context.

An important context in which psychotherapy and supervision are practised is the ethics and standards of professional practice. Discussing ethical dilemmas and reflecting on the standards of professional practice are vital supervision processes. Supervision has an important qualitative function, which ensures that the work of psychotherapy is provided ethically and professionally (Hawkins & Shohet, 2012).

Summary

In this chapter, we have described the development of MCIS, its fundamental principles, and the core processes of change in integrative supervision. Throughout the rest of the book, we will be referring to these fundamental principles and processes of change. In integrative supervision, all processes of change are essential, and we flexibly use all of them. However, this book focuses on change processes specific to our MCIS approach: Mindfulness and compassion processes and processes related to emotional and physiological regulation.

Chapter 2

Relating from the observing self

Mindfulness and compassion in supervision

During the last decades, mindfulness and compassion have become important concepts both in psychotherapy and mental health in general. Kabat-Zinn (1994) describes mindfulness as "paying attention in a particular way: On purpose, in the present moment and non-judgmentally" (p. 4). In mindfulness- and compassion-oriented integrative psychotherapy (MCIP), we define mindfulness as a process of accepting awareness of the present moment (G. Žvelc & Žvelc, 2021). In addition to mindfulness, the process of compassion has also attracted increasing clinical and research interest (Germer & Neff, 2013; P. Gilbert, 2009, 2010; Neff, 2003a, 2003b; Neff & Germer, 2013). P. Gilbert (2009) defines compassion as "basic kindness, with deep awareness of the suffering of oneself and of other living things, coupled with the wish and effort to relieve it" (p. xiii). Research shows significant benefits of both mindfulness and compassion for mental health (Cavicchioli et al., 2018; Farb et al., 2007, 2012; Ferrari et al., 2019; Goldberg et al., 2018; MacBeth & Gumley, 2012; Teper & Inzlicht, 2013; Teper et al., 2013). There is also an increasing body of research showing the benefits of mindfulness- and compassion-oriented interventions in clinical training. A systematic review of qualitative research regarding trainee therapists' experience of mindfulness training has shown several benefits for their personal and professional development, such as enhanced emotional regulation and well-being, stronger therapeutic relationships, and better boundaries between therapist and client (Fletcher et al., 2022). Mindfulness interventions may also positively affect the practice of psychotherapy through enhanced therapist empathy (Garrote-Caparrós et al., 2022). Compassion-focused interventions are related to the trainees' development of their capacities for emotional regulation and healthy coping strategies (Beaumont et al., 2017). They reduce self-criticism and promote self-compassion and compassion for others (Beaumont et al., 2017; Bell et al., 2017). Cultivation of self-compassion reduces worry and rumination and may increase self-reflection (Bell et al., 2017). It is suggested that self-compassion is also essential for trainees' self-care and prevention of burnout (Coaston, 2017; Nelson et al., 2018).

While there is now a vast amount of literature and research on mindfulness and compassion in psychotherapy, surprisingly little is written regarding mindfulness

DOI: 10.4324/9781003194118-4

and compassion in supervision. There are, however, some notable exceptions. Coaston (2019) proposes that cultivating self-compassion and mindfulness within the supervisory relationship may have several benefits for the clinician's professional development and demonstrates how self-compassion can be integrated into supervision. McCrea & Bulanda (2008) described the important role of compassion-based supervision for residential care staff, while Banker & Goldenson (2021) propose that using mindfulness in supervision produces many benefits for supervisees. Haberlin (2020) argues for the importance of mindfulness in supervision and proposes a model of mindfulness-based supervision. In his model, the central idea is that of the supervisor who develops mindful qualities and is present centred, aware of their thoughts and emotions and what is occurring in the environment. Based on the work of Kabat-Zinn (1990), he proposes that the supervisor develops seven attitudes of mindfulness: Non-judgement, patience, beginner's mind, trust, non-striving, acceptance, and letting go. Haberlin (2020) describes such a supervisor with the concept of an *awakened supervisor*.

In our previous work, we have proposed that mindfulness and compassion are core psychotherapy processes that can be enhanced by different methods within the attuned therapeutic relationship (G. Žvelc & Žvelc, 2021). Similarly to psychotherapy, in our approach to supervision (mindfulness- and compassion-oriented integrative supervision (MCIS)), mindfulness and compassion are viewed as core processes of supervision. This chapter describes the framework for integrating mindfulness and compassion in supervision, drawing from MCIP (G. Žvelc & Žvelc, 2021). We emphasise how MCIP models can be used in the supervision process (the diamond model of the observing self, the triangle of relationship to internal experience, and the keyhole model of relational mindfulness and compassion).

The diamond model of the observing self and supervision process

Figure 2.1 shows the diamond model of the observing self (G. Žvelc & Žvelc, 2021), which presents the observing self as a central concept related to mindful awareness and compassion.

Figure 2.1 presents the observing self as the sun with its rays (illustrated by arrows) "shining" towards different dimensions of human experience: Cognitive, affective, physiological, behavioural, and relational. The sun in the centre represents the observing self, and different rays describe the process of mindful awareness of different contents of experience. The figure symbolically presents the mindful awareness of both internal and external experiences. Mindful awareness of internal experiences refers to internal contact – accepting awareness of our thoughts, emotions, body, and behaviour. Figure 2.1 portrays this through the rays pointing to different dimensions in the square. Rays pointing to the circle portray our contact with other people

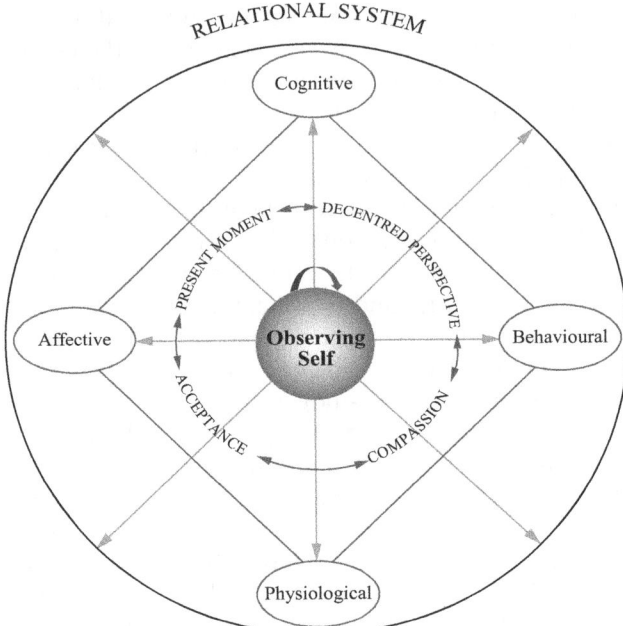

Figure 2.1 The diamond model of the observing self.

Note: Reprinted from *Integrative psychotherapy: A mindfulness- and compassion-oriented approach* (p. 40), by G. Žvelc & M. Žvelc, 2021, Routledge. Copyright 2021 by G. Žvelc & M. Žvelc. Reprinted with permission of the authors and the publisher (Taylor & Francis Ltd, www.tandfonline.com).

or the environment – external contact. The figure also includes an arrow pointing back at the observing self, representing awareness of the observing self (awareness of awareness).

The observing self is "our essential sense of self that is awareness itself" (G. Žvelc & Žvelc, 2021, p. 37). We have also described it as *self-as-awareness* (G. Žvelc & Žvelc, 2021), the aspect of ourselves from which we experience all our thoughts, emotions, sensations, and perceptions of the external environment. This sense of self is often described as "self-as-context" or "transcendent self" (S. C. Hayes et al., 2012). It is the context of all our experience that cannot itself be perceived as it is a perspective from which we perceive and experience. The observing self has transcendent qualities (Deikman, 1982) and can only be experienced and not grasped as an object of our perception.

In Figure 2.1, the observing self in the centre relates to the sense of awareness and presence ("I am aware"), while rays pointing to different dimensions describe the contents of awareness at a particular moment in time ("what I am aware of"). While the innermost centre (observing self) is constant and stable, the contents of experience are transient and changing. Our physical sensations, emotions, thoughts, and our perceptions of the external environment continually change; however, our sense of awareness is always there.

Qualities of the observing self and the supervision process

As we have described in our previous work, contact with the observing self is a source of psychological health and healing and has several benefits for both ourselves and other people (G. Žvelc & Žvelc, 2021). The observing self has the following qualities: Mindful awareness and presence, compassion, stable perspective, a container of experience, transcendence, and spirituality.

The observing self is a source of *mindful awareness and presence* and is subjectively experienced as a simple experience of *being* and conscious *presence*. In our supervision practice, we invite our supervisees to contact the observing self and relate to their inner experience with mindful awareness. That means they relate to their thoughts, emotions, and body sensations in the present moment, with acceptance and from a decentred perspective. We have found that this process is essential in supervision practice and has several benefits for the supervision process. Mindful awareness of the supervisee's inner experience leads to internal and external contact, brings insights, and promotes self-regulation and processing of experience. When supervisees start talking about their client, their relational schemas of being with that client are activated, bringing their experience and sense of the client into the supervision room. Mindful observation of their inner experience helps to bring insight about themselves, the client, and their relationship and illuminates the current relationship with the supervisor. Mindfulness also promotes self-regulation and processing of emotional experiences.

Contact with the observing self inherently brings *compassion*, either to self or others (S. C. Hayes et al., 2012; G. Žvelc & Žvelc, 2021). As our supervisees are often highly self-critical, self-compassion is a crucial process that helps supervisees to relate to themselves with love, acceptance, forgiveness, and understanding. In addition to self-compassion, we also invite supervisees to develop compassion for their clients. When supervisees can deeply experience the suffering of their clients and can observe that suffering from the position of the observing self, compassion naturally arises.

Relating from the observing self brings a *stable perspective* from which we can observe all our experiences. While our contents of awareness are transient and change, the observing self is always there and brings stability and safety. The observing self is the context of all our experiences, and we can describe it as a container in which all experiences arise (S. C. Hayes et al., 2012). When we invite our supervisees to contact their observing self, they can experience all their difficult moments related to their psychotherapeutic work from a stable and safe perspective. That helps them to contain, self-regulate, and process their experience.

The observing self has *transcendental qualities* (Deikman, 1982; S. C. Hayes, 1984; S. C. Hayes et al., 2012; G. Žvelc & Žvelc, 2021). It is the aspect of ourselves that cannot be perceived as an object but only experienced. In different spiritual traditions, it is described as *no-thing* self and *pure awareness* (S. C. Hayes et al., 1999, 2012). It can also be described as our *essential self* in contrast to our *personal self*, which refers to our identity (G. Žvelc & Žvelc, 2021). Awareness of the observing self may also result in an experience of non-dual awareness that is related to the experience of unity and inter-connection with other people and nature. While this is an important aim in different wisdom traditions, this is not usually the aim in psychotherapy or supervision practice. However, awareness of the observing self in supervision often brings mental health practitioners closer to their meaning and purpose and in touch with the spiritual dimension of their psyche.

Processes of mindfulness and compassion in supervision

From amongst the qualities of the observing self, we emphasise mindful awareness and compassion as the two core qualities that are crucial for the supervision process. Mindful awareness consists of three main processes: Present moment awareness, acceptance, and decentred perspective. As we describe in Chapter 1, we view these processes and the process of compassion as core meta-processes of supervision. They influence and enhance other change processes, such as emotional and physiological regulation, mentali-sation, awareness and acceptance of emotions, and interoception.

Figure 2.1 presents all four processes of mindful awareness and compas-sion illustrated within a circle that shows how all these processes are related to each dimension of human experience.

Present moment awareness

Present moment awareness is a crucial process of mindfulness. The inability to be in the present moment manifests in ruminations about the past or the future and a lack of awareness of certain aspects of inner experience or the external environment. Supervisees may, for example, become caught in pat-terns of unproductive worrying about themselves or their clients. Some su-pervisees are overconcerned with methodological aspects of therapeutic work while losing contact with themselves and the client. Supervisees may be unaware of their thoughts, emotions, body sensations, or behaviour. They may have problems being fully present with the client or supervisor.

By inviting our supervisees to the present moment, we enhance their ability to become fully aware of what is happening within themselves and in the supervisory relationship. By attending to their inner experience, they may become aware of emotions, thoughts, and body sensations related to the supervision or their therapy with clients. That enhances mentalisation and self-reflection. Contact with the present moment also helps supervisees to develop their ability for mindful and compassionate presence during a therapy session.

Acceptance

Acceptance is the second fundamental process of mindful awareness (G. Žvelc & Žvelc, 2021). It relates to openness and non-judgement of experience. By acceptance, we are embracing and allowing all our experiences, either pleasant or unpleasant. For mindfulness, present moment awareness is not enough; it must be coupled with the acceptance of experience (Černetič, 2017). The lack of acceptance manifests in avoidance of emotions, physical sensations, and thoughts – in experiential avoidance (S. C. Hayes et al., 2012). As with our clients, we as a therapist naturally avoid certain experiences that are too painful. In supervision, experiential avoidance often manifests in a supervisee's struggle to talk about certain experiences, over-intellectualisation, and lack of contact with their inner experiences. Some supervisees tend to speak very fast, which is often related to the control of certain feelings they are unwilling to experience. Avoidance of countertransference related to the specific client may impact the therapist's ability to form an effective relationship with them. For an effective relationship, the therapist must be in full contact with themselves and the client (Erskine, 2015). Chronic avoidance of inner experience may also negatively impact the therapist's health, leading to psychosomatic problems or burnout. In MCIS, we invite the supervisee to accept their experiences and reverse the cycle of experiential avoidance.

Decentred perspective

Decentred perspective is the third core process of mindful awareness (G. Žvelc & Žvelc, 2021). It relates to the ability to observe our experience without being merged with it. For mindful awareness, "differentiation between the I, who is aware, and the content of my experience" is crucial (G. Žvelc & Žvelc, 2021, p. 43). It helps us to *look at the experience* rather than *from the experience*. This means that we can observe our thoughts, emotions, and bodily sensations without being caught up in them or avoiding them. Metaphorically, it is as if we were standing by a river and observing the leaves on the water that come and go. This ability is crucial in supervision and enables practitioners to reflect upon their experiences. The opposite process is merging with experience, or as S. C. Hayes et al. (2012) describe it – cognitive fusion. In this case, the experience of I is identified with the contents of experience, which manifests in a lack of observational space and reflection. In the supervision process, this may be reflected in preoccupation with certain client's experiences, inability to let go of the client after the session, and ongoing rumination regarding the client. It may also be related to over-identification with the therapist's personal issues, such as lack of self-worth or shame. Enhancing a decentred perspective is, consequently, one of the important goals in the supervision process.

Compassion

In addition to the three processes of mindful awareness, compassion is another crucial process of supervision. As we have already described, compassion naturally arises when we can look at other people or ourselves through the eyes of the observing self. For compassion, all three previously described mindful processes are necessary: Present moment awareness, acceptance, and decentred perspective. While mindful awareness is directed towards a certain internal experience or outer perception, compassion is directed towards a person who suffers. Compassion involves the intention that a person in pain is relieved from their suffering (Gilbert, 2010).

In MCIS, we enhance both the self-compassion of the supervisee and compassion directed towards their clients. Neff (2003b, 2011) describes three main components of self-compassion: Self-kindness, common humanity, and mindfulness. Self-compassion brings kindness towards ourselves when experiencing pain and helps us to understand that our imperfections, pain, and suffering are all part of our shared human experience. In our experience, psychotherapists are often very critical and judgemental towards themselves and have difficulty relating to themselves with kindness and love. Whilst they may be thoroughly dedicated to their clients, they are often not treating themselves with the same level of respect and dignity. Psychotherapeutic work itself can often be stressful and painful for the psychotherapist. It is important that psychotherapists acknowledge this and treat themselves with compassion and care. Enhancing self-compassion helps psychotherapists develop a nurturing and loving inner relationship, a cornerstone of mental health and prevention against burnout. The loving inner relationship is beneficial in psychotherapy, as it brings a compassionate presence to the psychotherapy relationship. Such presence helps the supervisee to self-regulate, contain painful emotions, and relate with care to their clients.

The use of the diamond model of the observing self in supervision

The diamond model of the observing self is a model that has important clinical implications in both supervision and psychotherapy. The model is used for process diagnostics of mindfulness processes concerning the main dimensions of human experience: Cognitive, affective, physiological, behavioural, and relational. In supervision, the supervisor can assess the supervisee's ability to relate to each dimension with mindful awareness. If the supervisee lacks mindful awareness in relation to a particular dimension, the supervisor can encourage them to relate to that dimension with present moment awareness, decentred perspective, and acceptance. In MCIS, we use mindfulness- and compassion-oriented interventions directed to different dimensions of human experience: Cognitive, affective, physiological, behavioural, and relational. With the help of interventions based on mindful awareness, we expand the awareness and contact of the supervisee with different dimensions here and now. In Chapter 7, we describe various interventions that encourage the processes of mindful awareness related to these main dimensions of human experience.

The triangle of relationship to internal experience in supervision

In our previous work, we developed the triangle of relationship to internal experience model, which describes three primary relationships with phenomenological experience: 1) Being merged with the experience, 2) being distanced from the experience, and 3) being a loving witness to our experience (see Figure 2.2) (G. Žvelc & Žvelc, 2021). In supervision practice, the model helps us to evaluate the supervisee's level of mindful awareness and helps us to guide them towards contact with the observing self, the loving witness.

These three different relationships to internal experience are the result of the three different expressions of mindful processes: Present moment awareness, acceptance, and decentred perspective. Being merged and being distanced describe two different non-mindful ways of being, whereas loving witness is related to mindful awareness and is the quality of the observing self.

Loving witness
(high awareness, acceptance and decentred perspective)

Being distant   Being merged
(low awareness, high avoidance)   *(low awareness, high fusion)*

Figure 2.2 The triangle of relationship to internal experience.

Note: Reprinted from *Integrative psychotherapy: A mindfulness- and compassion-oriented approach* (p. 45), by G. Žvelc & M. Žvelc, 2021, Routledge. Copyright 2021 by G. Žvelc & M. Žvelc. Reprinted with permission of the authors and the publisher (Taylor & Francis Ltd, www.tandfonline.com).

Being merged with the experience

When supervisees are merged with their experience, they are often identified with their countertransference experience related to their clients. They have difficulties establishing a decentred perspective and are often overwhelmed with the client's problems and difficulties or their reactions towards them. When they are merged with their experience, this prevents them from effectively intervening and reflecting upon the therapeutic relationship. Extreme states of merging may manifest in overwhelming emotions and unproductive ruminations related to their clients. When supervisees are merged with their experience related to their clients, they also have problems being in the present moment and being aware of other options related to their work. If the states of merging remain for longer periods, this can also lead to exhaustion, burnout, and empathic distress. In qualitative research, which investigated the empathic distress of psychotherapists, it was found that the inability to keep an appropriate distance between themselves and their clients was the main contributor to empathic distress (Uršič & Žvelc, 2017).

In supervision practice, we help supervisees to decentre from their experience and observe in the present moment their experience with interest and curiosity. This helps them to disidentify from their experience and develop more internal space, which helps them to reflect upon their experience.

Being distanced from the experience

Being distanced from inner experience is the opposite extreme of being merged. It is another non-mindful way of being and experiencing the world. In this case, supervisees may be detached from their experience related to their clients. They may feel dull and empty and have difficulty being in contact with their inner experience. This manifests in an inability to be aware of their thoughts, emotions, or body sensations. In extreme cases, they may be dissociated. Being distanced from the experience is related to low awareness and avoidance of inner experience. In mindfulness- and compassion-oriented supervision, we aim for full contact with the experience and invite our supervisees to gradually come into contact with their experience. In this case, we invite them to be fully aware of their experiences related to their clients and invite them to fully accept whatever they feel. Interventions related to the present moment awareness of bodily sensations and their acceptance are primary in the case of distance from inner experience.

Being a loving witness to our experience

Being a loving witness to our experience is shown in Figure 2.2, portrayed at the top of the triangle, and represents the ability to relate to our experience in the present moment, with acceptance and from a decentred perspective. This is the paramount quality of the observing self and enables effective self-reflection, openness, and contact with the experience. In this position, we are also open to new learning. We believe such a relationship to inner experience is central to effective supervision and psychotherapy. It helps us to reflect on our experience of both therapeutic and supervisory relationships. It is the supervisor's primary position, and their task in MCIS is to invite the supervisee to relate to their experience from the position of the loving witness. The word "loving" is related to openness and acceptance of all our experiences, both pleasant and unpleasant. It is not a cold, intellectual, detached observation. With the concept of a loving witness, we want to imply full contact with experience that is characterised by kindness, warmth, and openness towards all of our experiences.

In supervision, we help supervisees to move from the non-mindful positions of merging or distance to the position of a loving witness, which enables contact, reflection, and new learning in supervision.

The keyhole model of relational mindfulness and compassion in supervision

In MCIS, we have developed several interventions and methods that invite the supervisee to relate to their experience from the perspective of the loving witness – observing self. Different chapters of this book describe various ways in which mindfulness and compassion can be used in the supervision process. Central to all these interventions are methods of relational mindfulness and compassion related to the keyhole model of relational mindfulness and compassion (see Figure 2.3) (G. Žvelc & Žvelc, 2021). The model integrates Erskine's *keyhole model* (Erskine et al., 1999, 2023) with processes of mindfulness and compassion. The main assumption of this model is that mindfulness and compassion can be most effectively used in psychotherapy and supervision within an attuned relationship. While most mindfulness approaches focus on mindfulness and compassion as a technique to be learned by the client or therapist, we emphasise the importance of bringing mindfulness and compassion to the heart of the supervisory relationship. In MCIS, we give importance to mindful awareness of both supervisor and supervisee. The fundamental principle is that "two aware minds are more powerful than only one" (G. Žvelc, 2012, p. 47). The mindful and compassionate presence of the supervisor is like a catalyst for the supervisees' mindful awareness and compassion. The supervisees' mindful awareness and compassion are then transferred back to their relationship with their clients (see Chapter 3).

The keyhole model of relational mindfulness and compassion illustrates how mindfulness and compassion can be encouraged by the three core methods of integrative psychotherapy: *Inquiry, attunement, and involvement*

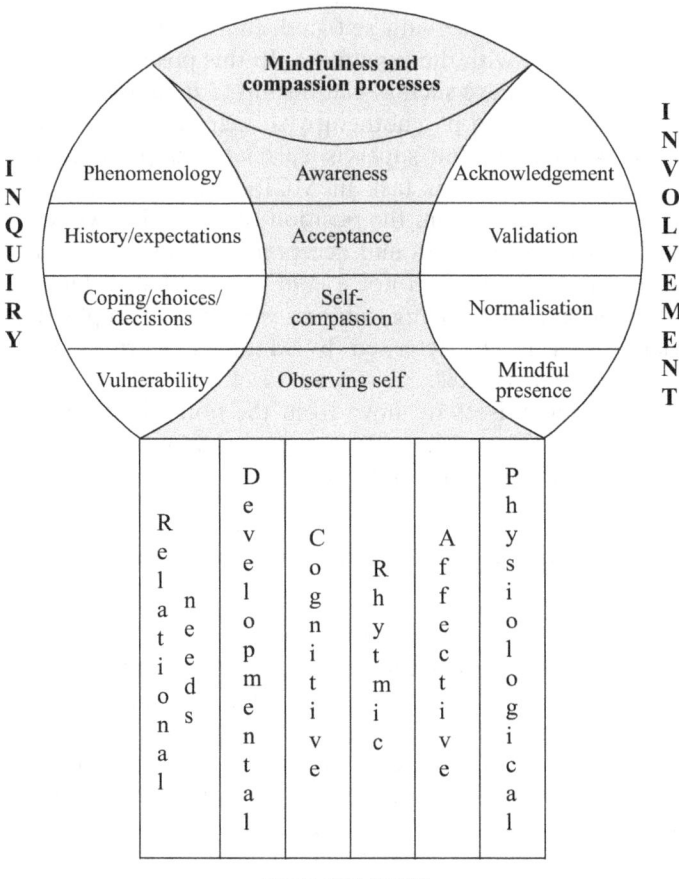

ATTUNEMENT

Figure 2.3 Keyhole model of relational mindfulness and compassion.

Note: Reprinted from Integrative Psychotherapy: A mindfulness- and compassion-oriented approach (p. 40), by G. Žvelc & M. Žvelc, 2021, Routledge. The figure is adapted from Beyond Empathy: A therapy of contact-in-relationship (p. 159), by R. G. Erskine, J. P. Moursund, and R. L. Trautmann, 1999, Brunner/Mazel. Copyright 2021 by G. Žvelc & M. Žvelc. Reprinted with permission of the authors and the publisher (Taylor & Francis Ltd, www.tandfonline.com).

(Erskine et al., 1999, 2023; G. Žvelc & Žvelc, 2021). These relational methods are also essential in our supervision model and encourage supervisees to come into contact with the observing self and relate to their experience from the position of a loving witness. Inquiry, attunement, and involvement enhance core mindful awareness and compassion processes: Awareness of the present moment, decentred perspective, acceptance, and compassion (G. Žvelc & Žvelc, 2021).

Phenomenological inquiry

Erskine (1993) describes inquiry as a "respectful exploration of the client's phenomenological experience" (p. 186). Phenomenological inquiry is a fundamental intervention in MCIS that invites the supervisee to come into present moment awareness. It invites the supervisee to explore their experience, which helps them to become increasingly aware of their internal processes. Inquiry involves the ability to decentre from preconceived ideas and instead bring curiosity and genuine interest in the relationship (Erskine, 2015). It involves the ability of the supervisor to make an open space for the supervisee's experience and, at the same time, be fully present and in contact with themselves. Inquiry involves sensitive questions and statements that invite the supervisee to explore their experience in relation to their client or supervisor. It also involves non-verbal communication, such as tone of voice and facial expressions, that communicate genuine interest in knowing another person's experience (Erskine et al., 2023). Inquiry is related to all the main dimensions of human experience: Cognitive, affective, physiological, behavioural, and relational. The inquiry also promotes mentalisation and self-reflection, which are among the main factors of successful supervision.

Involvement

The supervisor not only explores the supervisee's experience but provides an involved response. Involvement is an expression of the person's full internal and external contact (Erskine et al., 2023). Involvement is conveyed by *acknowledgement*, *validation*, and *normalisation* of another person's experience (Erskine et al., 2023). These interventions, combined with the supervisor's *mindful presence*, enhance the supervisee's present moment awareness, acceptance, and self-compassion.

With *acknowledgement*, the supervisor communicates that they are aware of the supervisee's experience or behaviour. Acknowledgement goes hand in hand with phenomenological inquiry, as both interventions promote awareness of the present moment. With *validation*, the supervisor conveys to the supervisee that their experience is significant and valuable and promotes acceptance of the experience. *Normalisation* de-pathologises the person's definition of their inner experiences or coping mechanisms (Erskine, 2015). Normalisation conveys to the supervisee that their experience is a normal and not pathological reaction. It enhances the process of self-compassion, as it is related to a sense of common humanity – that all our experiences are part of being human.

The fourth aspect of involvement is *mindful presence*, which refers to the supervisor's way of being (G. Žvelc & Žvelc, 2021). In the MCIS approach, the cultivation of mindful presence is essential for the supervision process. The supervisor's mindful presence helps the supervisor relate to themselves and the supervisee from the position of a loving witness. This involves the ability to recognise thoughts, emotions, and physical sensations related to the supervision process, as well as mindful observation of the supervisee's non-verbal reactions. It involves the ability to look at ourselves and others from a decentred compassionate perspective. The mindful presence of the supervisor pervades all other interventions of the supervisor, which are conveyed with mindful sensitivity, genuine interest, acceptance of the other person's experience, and welfare for the well-being of the supervisee and their clients. The supervisor's presence may be a catalyst for the supervisee's mindful presence.

Attunement

Attunement is the third relational method that provides the foundation for all other methods and interventions in the supervision process and is crucial for developing an effective supervisory relationship. Erskine & Trautmann (1996) describe attunement as a "kinesthetic and emotional sensing of the other – knowing his or her rhythm, affect, and experience by metaphorically being in his or her skin, thus going beyond empathy to provide a reciprocal affect and/ or resonating response" (p. 320). Erskine et al. (1999) described five aspects of attunement: Cognitive, affective, rhythmic, developmental, and attunement to relational needs. To these five aspects, we have added the sixth aspect of attunement – physiological attunement, which is crucial for physiological regulation (G. Žvelc & Žvelc, 2021).

In supervision, the goal of attunement is to establish an effective supervisory relationship, which provides the foundation for the use of mindfulness- and compassion-oriented interventions. Attunement also potentiates mindful awareness, as attunement to the supervisee's experience raises awareness of their cognitive processes, emotions, relational needs, and physiological processes. The supervisor's attunement is like a beam of light that brings awareness to the supervisee's experience, which is often non-verbalised, implicit, and very subtle. Through the supervisor's non-verbal attuned and compassionate response, the supervisee comes into touch with themselves and may start to relate to themselves with openness, acceptance, and self-compassion.

Attunement also helps us to understand the implicit, unconscious communication between the supervisee and supervisor that may be transferred from psychotherapy to the supervisory relationship – the parallel process. We explore the parallel process in detail in Chapter 3.

Cognitive attunement helps us to deeply understand the supervisee's frame of reference and helps us to uncover implicit communication that is behind the supervisee's verbal narratives. By attuning to the supervisee's use of words and logical reasoning, we may also intuit the possible parallel process stemming from the therapeutic relationship to the supervisory relationship.

Affective attunement involves empathic sensing of another person's affect and responding with reciprocal affect (Erskine & Trautmann, 1996). The supervisor may, for example, respond to the supervisee's fear and anxiety by providing stability and security. Affective attunement provides a reciprocal attuned response that helps to regulate the supervisee's emotions. Such emotional regulation is then transferred back to the primary therapeutic relationship.

Rhythmic attunement in supervision helps us to attune to another person's rhythm and facilitates optimal processing of both internal and external stimuli (Erskine & Trautmann, 1996). To facilitate mindfulness and compassion, supervisees must pause and take time to come into touch with themselves. Rhythmic attunement in MCIS is often related to slowing down the pace of the supervision, which enables supervisees to be with their experience with openness and curiosity. This also helps to regulate the supervisee's emotions and autonomic nervous system.

Developmental attunement in supervision is related to understanding and responding to the supervisee's developmental level in terms of their professional development. For example, supervisees at an early stage may need more confidence building and skill development, while supervisees at a more advanced stage may need more focus on multi-theoretical perspectives (Erskine, 1982). There is another meaning of developmental attunement: Attunement to archaic self-states manifesting in the supervision process. As our clients, our supervisees often react from child self-states related to previous developmental phases when certain traumatic events may have occurred. Through developmental attunement, the supervisor may detect these younger parts of the supervisee and make them explicit through attuned and involved response. Through this process, the supervisor and supervisee uncover the personal issues that may have been reactivated in the supervisee. The archaic child self-states of supervisees that manifest in supervision are often related to the dynamics of the client–therapist relationship. By uncovering the supervisee's self-states, we may better understand the psychotherapy process.

Attunement to relational needs is also an essential aspect of attunement and refers to the supervisor's relational style that is flexible to the current needs of the supervisee emerging in the course of supervision. By attunement to relational needs, supervisees become aware of their needs in supervision or in their relationship with their clients (Stewart, 2010).

Erskine (2015) developed the model of relational needs that are not only important in psychotherapy but are essential to all human relationships. Relational needs can only be satisfied in an attuned and involved human relationship (Erskine, 2015). These needs are present throughout life, from infancy to old age. G. Žvelc et al. (2020) have validated Erskine's model in empirical research and found five primary relational needs: 1) Authenticity, 2) support and protection, 3) having an impact, 4) shared experience, and 5) initiative from the other. The model was further confirmed in empirical studies in Spain, Czechia, and Turkey (Iraurgi et al., 2022; Pourová et al., 2020; Toksoy et al., 2020). As in other relationships, relational needs are also essential in the supervisory relationship. Attunement to relational needs in supervision means that the supervisor responds appropriately according to the relational needs that emerge in the supervisory relationship. If the *need for authenticity* is in the foreground, the supervisor may value the uniqueness of the supervisee's style of work and encourage them to develop their own way of being as a therapist. Sometimes, the supervisee needs *support and protection* from the supervisor, especially when they feel vulnerable or threatened by the client. This is especially important when working with difficult clients, such as suicidal clients (M. Žvelc, 2017). When the *need for having an impact* is uppermost, the supervisor may show that they are affected by the supervisee. This shows either in their interest in the supervisees' ideas and thinking or in sharing their emotional response to the supervisee. When the *need for shared experience* is in the foreground, the supervisor may share experiences from their own therapeutic practice that are similar to what happened to the supervisee. If supervision occurs in the group context, this need is best responded to by group members sharing their own experiences similar to the supervisee's experiences.

G. Žvelc & Žvelc (2021) also described the sixth aspect of attunement, *physiological attunement*, that is essential in MCIS. Physiological attunement is attunement to the supervisee's arousal of their autonomic nervous system. It refers to sensing the physiological arousal of the supervisee and providing the corresponding response. The supervisor synchronises with the autonomic nervous system of the supervisee or regulates it if the supervisee is in a state of physiological dysregulation. If the supervisee's autonomic nervous system is in the optimal arousal zone, then the supervisor's adaptive response is physiological synchronisation with the supervisee. If the supervisee is dysregulated in either hyperarousal or hypoarousal, the supervisor's task is to stop the dysfunctional synchronisation and take the lead towards physiological regulation and the optimal arousal zone.

Compared to psychotherapy, methods of relational mindfulness and compassion in supervision differ in their goals. While the goal in psychotherapy is contact and reintegration of long-forgotten and dissociated parts of the client, the goals in supervision are related primarily to the tasks and goals of the supervision process. And so, in contrast to psychotherapy, we usually do not explore past issues of the supervisee. Occasionally, we may ask the supervisee to connect their experience with their past issues, which provides an understanding of their countertransference response. The goal, however, is not integration and processing of the supervisee's past unresolved issues. In supervision, we may identify them and encourage the supervisee to work on them in their personal psychotherapy. In supervision, we mainly use phenomenological inquiry and involvement that are related to exploring the supervisor's experience and reflections in relation to their psychotherapy work.

From supervision to clinical practice and daily life

An invitation to relate from the position of the observing self in supervision brings benefits not only within the supervision setting, but also has important benefits for clinical practice and daily life. When we invite our supervisees to relate from the observing self, they will gradually develop the capacity to relate to their clients with mindful presence and compassion. Supervision is a "training space" for supervisees' clinical practice and daily life. By bringing mindful interventions into the supervision process, the supervisor models how to apply them in therapy. The supervisee internalises mindful interventions of the supervisor and then uses them in their own therapy sessions. We suggest that the supervisor applies all the processes of mindfulness and compassion to themselves as they are also helpful for the supervisor's mental health and prevention of burnout. The qualities of the observing self are not only important in our professional context but also in our everyday life. They help practitioners to bring mindful awareness and compassion to themselves and others.

Summary

We have described three main models crucial for assessing mindfulness and compassion in supervision and tailoring effective clinical interventions. The diamond model of the observing self helps us to understand and assess the supervisee's mindful awareness and compassion related to different personality dimensions: Cognitive, affective, physiological, behavioural, and relational. If the supervisee lacks mindful awareness in relation to a particular dimension, the supervisor can encourage mindful awareness concerning that particular dimension.

The triangle of relationship to internal experience helps us decide which process of mindful awareness is crucial to encourage. If the supervisee is merged with their experience, interventions that promote present moment awareness and decentred perspective will be most helpful. Similarly, if the supervisee is distanced from their experience, then interventions that invite the supervisee to contact their experience in the present moment with acceptance will be central.

The keyhole model of relational mindfulness and compassion is the model of clinical interventions related to mindfulness and compassion. It helps us to understand which interventions can be used to promote present moment awareness, decentred perspective, acceptance, and compassion. These three models are the cornerstone of MCIS, and in later chapters of this book, we relate to these models and show how mindful awareness and compassion can be encouraged in supervision.

Chapter 3

Mindfulness- and compassion-oriented transformative supervision model

Mindfulness- and compassion-oriented integrative supervision (MCIS) is an integrative supervision approach based on multiple pathways of change in supervision. The primary model specific to our approach is the mindfulness- and compassion-oriented transformative supervision model (MCIS transformative model). It explains how the changes in MCIS occur. The core assumption of this model is that mindfulness and compassion processes in supervision transform the supervisee's way of being and their relational schemas of being with the client. While our approach uses different interventions that focus on all classical supervision tasks, we give special attention to mindfulness and compassion interventions that aim to transform the supervisee's emotional and body experience.

Supervisees often experience complex emotional and physiological states in their work as psychotherapists and struggle to regulate them. Sometimes they may be unaware of the presence of these dysregulated physiological or emotional states. Dysregulated experiences are stored in dysfunctional relational schemas of being with the client and influence subsequent interaction with the client, the therapist's personal life, and the supervision process.

Processes of mindfulness, compassion, and emotional and physiological regulation help transform the supervisee's dysregulated experiences and bring new insights and understanding of self, client, and their relationship. In this way, supervision provides new experiences needed to change the relational schemas of being with the client. With the help of supervision, supervisees enter their subsequent psychotherapy sessions with a new experience of themselves and the client. After supervision, they often feel more present and compassionate in psychotherapy sessions. This also enhances therapists' mentalisation ability and helps them to think and respond more flexibly. The psychotherapist's transformed way of being also has numerous benefits for their well-being and helps to prevent burnout.

The MCIS model can be summarised in the following way:

1   Development of relational schemas of being with the client.

DOI: 10.4324/9781003194118-5

2 Transformation of dysfunctional schemas and development of new relational schemas.
3 A new relationship with the client.

Development of relational schemas of being with the client

Relational schemas are schemas of a person's subjective experience of a relationship (G. Žvelc, 2009). They are generalisations of repeated experiences with other people and represent prototypes of relational events (G. Žvelc, 2010; G. Žvelc & Žvelc, 2021). The term relational schema entails not only verbal beliefs about self and others, but also the nonverbal implicit elements that include emotions, body sensations, and body movements (G. Žvelc, 2009). Relational schemas include the totality of an individual's experience of being with another person and include all dimensions of a person's experience: Cognitive, emotional, physiological, and behavioural (G. Žvelc, 2009).

Relational schemas are the lenses through which we look at ourselves and other people. They "affect the way we establish interpersonal relationships and how we relate to ourselves" (G. Žvelc & Žvelc, 2021, p. 73). Activation of schemas influences how we perceive, interpret, and react towards another person. This often occurs unconsciously. An individual may experience certain emotions and physical sensations and react in a specific way without realising that they are reacting based on past relational patterns stored in the relational schema.

Although our core relational schemas are developed in early childhood, we form relational schemas specific to other relationships throughout life (G. Žvelc, 2009). For psychotherapists, this is seen in relational schemas of being with their clients. These schemas are representations of being with a specific client and represent the therapist's experience of the client and their interaction.

Therapist's experience of being with the client and the concept of countertransference

An important concept in supervision is the concept of countertransference, coming from psychoanalysis. There exist many different views on countertransference, which often causes confusion. In the early days of psychoanalysis, countertransference was mainly understood as related to unresolved personal issues of the therapist, while later authors (Racker, 1968) understood countertransference also as an important tool for understanding the client. Maroda (2004) views countertransference as a totality of the therapist's reactions to the client. She defines it as "the conscious and unconscious responses of the therapist to the patient" (Maroda, 2004, p. 66). In this view, countertransference is not necessarily related to unprocessed and unresolved issues of the psychotherapist but is also a reaction towards a here-and-now experience with the client. These two aspects are interrelated and cannot be clearly distinguished to describe what is "real" and what is imaginary (Maroda, 2004).

In our mindfulness- and compassion-oriented integrative psychotherapy approach, we view phenomena that are attributed to the concept of transference and countertransference through the theory of relational schemas (G. Žvelc, 2009, 2010; G. Žvelc & Žvelc, 2021). Instead of the term countertransference, we often use the term *therapist's experience of being with the client*, which covers all of the psychotherapist's experiences and reactions related to their client. This includes the therapist's emotions, thoughts, physical sensations, and behaviour. From the perspective of relational schemas theory, the therapist's experience of being with the client is based on the therapist's previous relational schemas and their current experience with the client. These two aspects are intertwined. Each experience of being with the client includes elements related to the psychotherapist's past and their reactions to the client's current experience and behaviour. The concept of physiological synchrony describes how the therapist may synchronise with their client's physiology (see Chapter 4). The therapist may "feel" emotions and physiological states related to the client's experience. In this way, the therapist's experience of the client carries important information about the client.

The therapist's experience of the client is recorded in the relational schema of being with that client. For example, psychotherapist Peter felt fear in his relationship with his client and perceived him as very strict and controlling. The therapist, trying to please the client, did not confront him, even though the client was violating the boundaries of the client–therapist relationship (not coming on time, being late, not paying regularly). The experience of fear and adapting to the client was recorded in the relational schema of being with that client, which influenced subsequent psychotherapy sessions. The experience of fear and submission to the client was present in almost every therapeutic session.

Relational schemas can be either adaptive or dysfunctional (G. Žvelc & Žvelc, 2021). In the case of Peter, he developed a dysfunctional schema of their interaction, hindering the psychotherapeutic process. We can argue that Peter's fearful and submissive reaction resulted from his early relational schemas, maybe with his father or other significant people in his life. However, his experience in therapy was also influenced by the current dynamics with the client. It was the result of the interaction between his previous relational schemas and his current client experience. As G. Žvelc (2009) describes, when schemas are activated, this represents a re-awakening of past experience and, simultaneously, a new experience that a person has never had in the same form. Based on that, a new schema is developed, specific to the particular client–therapist relationship.

The relational schema includes important information about the therapist, the client, and their relationship. Such relational schemas may influence subsequent interaction with the client. If schemas are adaptive, they are flexible and open to change. The therapist, in this case, may react flexibly in a relationship with the client and can manage and contain their emotional experience. However, if the therapist cannot tolerate or regulate their physiological or emotional response, a dysfunctional schema may form. This schema will influence succeeding therapy sessions with the client and the therapist may become caught in repetitive patterns that are unproductive for psychotherapy progress. Supervision is a way to resolve such difficulties in psychotherapy and transform dysfunctional schemas.

Transformation of dysfunctional schemas and development of new relational schemas

In successful supervision, the supervisee's experience of being with the client is transformed, which has the potential to change dysfunctional relational schemas of being with their client. In addition to the transformation of dysfunctional schemas, supervision may also promote the development of new adaptive relational schemas of being with the supervisor. These processes are often intertwined and positively impact the supervisee's way of being with the client.

Supervision as a transformational process: The transformation of relational schemas of being with the client

When the supervisee starts discussing a certain client, the corresponding relational schema of being with that client is activated. The context of supervision is a stimulus that inevitably activates relational schemas of being with the client. The basic assumption of the MCIS transformative model is that dysfunctional relational schemas of being with the client can be transformed in supervision through the process of memory reconsolidation (Ecker et al., 2012). Physiological regulation, mindfulness, and compassion processes help transform the supervisee's dysregulated experience of the client and their relational schemas. The supervisor helps the supervisee transform them with mindfulness and compassion-oriented methods that provide new experiences that are contrary to their dysfunctional relational schema.

In MCIS, we intentionally bring awareness to activated relational schemas by inquiring the supervisee about their bodily felt experience of being with their client. While the supervisee's narrative about their client is important, we pay special attention to implicit elements of schemas that are felt in the body. More than in verbal narratives, we are interested in the implicit story communicated in bodily sensations, physical reactions, and emotions that underlie the verbal narrative. When relational schemas are activated, the relational experience of being with the client is re-awakened. The supervisee may experience self-states that reflect their experience of the client. Such self-states are manifested in bodily sensations, emotions, thoughts, and behaviour related to their clients. In the case of Peter, the supervisor invited him to pay attention to his body sensations while thinking about the client. Peter reported a terrible feeling in his stomach, which he identified as fear of the client. This helped him gain insight into the interactional pattern with his client and opened a further way for schema transformation.

When schemas are activated, they are open for transformational change through the process of memory reconsolidation (Ecker et al., 2012; Lane et al., 2015). Ecker (2015) describes memory reconsolidation as the "brain's innate process for fundamentally revising an existing learning and acquired behavioural responses and/or state of mind maintained by that learning" (p. 4). Through the process of memory reconsolidation, implicit emotional schemas can be revised at the level of "physical, neural synapses that encode it in emotional memory" (Ecker et al., 2012, p. 13).

For memory reconsolidation, it is necessary that relational schemas are activated and that the supervisee has a new experience that is juxtaposed with old learning. Dysfunctional schemas are transformed by repeated juxtapositional experiences between old and new learning. In MCIS, we intentionally bring awareness to implicit elements of activated schemas and make them open for change. Relational schemas of being with the client are developmentally newer schemas and are usually easier to change than dysfunctional schemas that stem from early childhood experiences. There are different ways to change schemas, and in integrative supervision, we may use multiple approaches for schema change. For example, a new relational experience with their supervisor may be an important new experience that counters a dysfunctional relational schema of being with the client. In MCIS, we specifically focus on the use of mindfulness and compassion for transformational changes in dysfunctional schemas. As we have described in our previous work (G. Žvelc & Žvelc, 2021), mindfulness and compassion processes are important pathways for schema change. They provide fundamentally new experiences in contrast to dysfunctional schemas – the experience of present moment awareness, acceptance, decentred perspective, and compassion. The book's second part describes specific methods and interventions that help transform dysfunctional schemas through mindfulness and self-compassion. In the case of Peter, the supervisor used a method of mindful processing, which helped to process the experience of fear and submission that he felt in his relationship with his client. At the end of this process, Peter experienced a sense of strength and self-confidence that was new to his relational schema, which had previously been dominated by a sense of inadequacy, submission, and fear of the client. The supervision experience helped him come to the next psychotherapy session with a different state of being, which involved self-respect and confidence. His physiology and emotions were regulated and within the window of tolerance. That made him feel more grounded and present in future psychotherapy sessions and enabled him to establish more clear boundaries with his client.

Our aim in MCIS is not only to empower the supervisee with new understanding and methodological knowledge but to affect change at the bodily/emotional level, which has the potential for transformation of implicit relational schemas of being with the client. The goal is for the supervisee to feel differently in supervision and their psychotherapy sessions and not just think or behave differently. In other words, in addition to influencing supervisees with "what to do" in their psychotherapy, we also influence "their way of being" in the therapy (S. M. Geller & Greenberg, 2012).

Development of new relational schemas of being with the supervisor/supervisory group

Supervision is a place where new learning occurs. Besides factual knowledge, supervisees acquire new ways of relating with themselves and others. They develop new skills and abilities such as self-awareness, self-reflection, and emotional and physiological regulation in the relationship. In MCIS, we are focused on developing mindful awareness and self-compassion abilities. One of the most important abilities in our approach is the supervisee's ability to recognise and regulate their level of physiological arousal. Supervisees in supervision gain new relational experiences with the supervisor and/or supervisory group. These new relational experiences are stored in relational schemas of being with the supervisor/supervisory group. These schemas provide a treasure of implicit relational knowing (Lyons-Ruth et al., 1998) that supervisees subsequently bring to their therapy sessions.

The concept of relational schemas of being with the supervisor is similar to Watkins' (2018a) concept of "Supervisee's Internal Representations of the Supervisor" (p. 64). Watkins (2018a) describes how supervisees form representations of their supervisor and that this can be an important facilitative educational factor relevant across different supervision approaches. Representations of the supervisor "involve the supervisee holding in mind the supervisor, or some aspects of the supervisor" (Watkins, 2018a, p. 66). Such representations involve internalisation of a supervisory dialogue and may include "the supervisor's attitude or way of being; statements that offer guidance and direction in moments of uncertainty; statements that express support for and belief in the therapist; and actions that are instructive and helpful with the treatment" (Watkins, 2018a, p. 66). If supervision is facilitative, these representations positively impact the client's treatment and the personal development of the therapist (J. D. Geller et al., 2010; Watkins, 2018a). Our concept of implicit relational schemas of being with the supervisor is similar to Watkins' (2018a) concept of representation; however, our concept specifically addresses the implicit affective and bodily components of representational structures.

We propose that relational schemas of being with the supervisor have a significant role in the development of the "internal supervisor" (Casement, 1985, 1990, 2002). Casement (1985, 1990) describes how the supervisee internalises aspects of the supervisory process and supervisory relationship and develops an internal dialogue during subsequent therapy, which acts as self-support and self-monitoring. Internal supervision is a process in which the therapist from moment-to-moment monitors what happens in the therapy session, observes, chooses, and evaluates different options of responding (Casement, 2002). Many supervision authors describe the development of an internal supervisor as one of the primary goals in the supervision process (M. C. Gilbert & Evans, 2000; Hawkins & Shohet, 2012). In MCIS, we specifically focus on developing *a mindful and compassionate internal supervisor*, which is then seen in the therapists' capacities for a mindful and compassionate stance towards self and the client. MCIS helps the supervisee develop the ability to be present in the therapy session and observe both self and the client with acceptance and compassion. This is congruent with the research of Bell et al. (2017), who found that compassion-focused interventions help therapists develop a compassionate internal supervisor, which shows in the decentred compassionate perspective towards self, others, and the therapeutic relationship.

In supervision, in addition to transforming the supervisee's dysfunctional schemas of being with the client, new relational schemas of being with the supervisor are developed. These schemas are an important resource in psychotherapy that helps the therapist to sustain mindful awareness and self-compassion and regulate themselves, even if dysfunctional relational schemas are activated. In some cases, the supervisee's experience of the client is influenced by their dysfunctional relational schemas related to past unresolved traumatic experiences. In such cases, relational schemas of being with the client are much more resistant to change as they are related to therapists' previously unprocessed issues. Mindfulness and compassion-oriented methods in supervision may not change such dysfunctional schemas but may provide what Ecker et al. (2012) call "counter-active" change. In supervision, a new relational schema is developed that copes with the activation of dysfunctional schema. For example, the supervisor helps to regulate a supervisee's particular emotional and physiological experience. Based on that, a new schema is formed that includes the experience of emotional and physiological regulation. The supervisee brings this new implicit knowledge of self-regulation to their next psychotherapy session. Even if their dysfunctional schemas are activated in the psychotherapeutic relationship, the supervisee has developed a new way of being that involves mindful awareness and compassion and can regulate their unbalanced physiology or emotion in the therapy. That frees up the reflective space that is essential for effective psychotherapy. New adaptive relational schemas of being with the supervisor, therefore, have an important role as a resource for coping with the activation of unresolved personal issues of the supervisee. Where such unresolved personal issues are present, further personal therapy of the supervisee is essential. The supervisor's task is to identify unresolved experiences related to past dysfunctional schemas and encourage the supervisee to deal with those issues in their own personal therapy.

The new relationship with the client

As we described in the previous section, supervision aims to transform the supervisee's experience of being with their client, which shows in transformed emotions, body-felt experience, and new understanding regarding the client, themselves, and their relationship. Through new experiences in supervision, dysfunctional relational schemas of being with the client are transformed through the process of memory reconsolidation. After supervision, the supervisee's way of being is changed. They often feel more present and compassionate to themselves and the client. Their emotions and physiology are regulated, and they are more in contact with their body and emotions. They have a new understanding regarding the self, the client, and the therapy relationship. The changed relational schema of being with the client affects their subsequent interactions with the client. Supervisees enter the following sessions with the client with regulated physiology, enabling them to bring mindful presence and compassion to the relationship with their client. This helps supervisees to form a new relationship with the client.

As we also described in the previous section, in addition to the transformation of dysfunctional schemas of being with the client, supervisees develop new relational schemas of being with their supervisor. Supervisees then bring their implicit learning of mindfulness and compassion from supervision to the therapy sessions. This enables them to relate to themselves and their clients with decentred perspective, acceptance, and compassion. Both dysfunctional schemas' transformations and new schemas' development help supervisees become more psychologically flexible. Psychological flexibility is one of the most important abilities related to psychological health and is related to full contact with the present moment and behaviour related to a person's chosen values (S. C. Hayes et al., 2012). Psychological flexibility enables the therapist to stay in contact with the present moment even though they may experience unpleasant thoughts, emotions, and body sensations while they choose interventions that are in the client's best interest.

In the case of the supervisee, Peter, he started to feel more grounded and present in psychotherapy with his client after a few supervision sessions. He reported that he felt differently, feeling more secure and calm. His physiology was regulated and in the optimal arousal zone. This enabled him to address issues with his client regarding boundary issues openly and respectfully. This change was also manifested in the supervisory relationship. Peter felt more open to suggestions from the supervisor, and the supervisor felt more grounded and secure. Both the psychotherapy relationship and supervisory relationship changed.

Implicit relational schemas, physiological synchrony, and the parallel process

The MCIS transformative model is influenced by the concept of the parallel process, which has its roots in psychoanalysis. Searles (1955) is recognised as the first author to write about the parallel process (Mothersole, 1999; Watkins, 2012). He described it as a *reflection process* in which "the processes at work currently in the relationship between patient and therapist are often reflected in the relationship between therapist and supervisor" (Searles, 1955, p. 135). He explained that the foundation of the parallel process is unconscious identification with the client and that supervisees are often unconsciously trying to tell the supervisor about the problem in the therapy. The supervisor's countertransferential emotional experience may be a reflection of what occurs in the client–therapist relationship or the client themself.

Watkins (2012) argues that the concept of parallel process is often defined vaguely. He suggests that we need a meaningful empirical definition of the parallel process that would be consistent, measurable, and have explanatory power. Tracey et al. (2012) conducted significant research on the parallel process where they defined the parallel process as bi-directional:

1   The therapist brings the interactional pattern between the therapist and the client into supervision and enacts the client's role.
2   The supervisee then takes the interactive pattern from the supervision back to the therapy session and enacts the supervisor's role.

The connection between both processes (in therapy and supervision) is the supervisee/therapist. Tracey et al. (2012) describe how the interactional pattern from supervision is taken back into the psychotherapy session. The parallel process does not involve only transmission from the psychotherapy session to the supervision process but also the other way around, with what happens in the supervision process being mirrored back in the psychotherapy relationship. This is what creates the opportunity for supervision to affect the psychotherapy relationship implicitly and automatically. The MCIS model is based on this idea and considers the transformative nature of supervision, which can also implicitly affect the psychotherapy relationship.

In MCIS, we understand the parallel process in supervision through the concept of relational schemas and physiological synchronisation. When the supervisee starts discussing a specific client, relational schemas of being with the client are activated in the supervisory relationship. Similar emotional and physiological states may occur in supervision as in psychotherapy with that client. The supervisee may re-experience thoughts, emotions, and physical sensations related to the client. Activated relational schemas of being with the client may also affect the way the supervisee experiences the supervisor and supervisory group members and are often the cause of ruptures in the supervisory alliance.

Relational schemas have two interrelated poles: The schema of the self and the schema of the other person (G. Žvelc, 2010). Supervisees may either enact in supervision the schema of self, which means that they bring and enact in supervision their role as a therapist, or they may enact the role of the client (schema of other). In supervision, they may repeat from the therapy session either 1) the perceived behaviour/state of mind of the client or 2) their own behaviour/state of mind. This process is often automatic, and supervisees are generally unaware that they are repeating the dynamics of the therapy session in the supervisory relationship. They may, for example, feel anxious and talk rapidly like their client or they may be detached and cold as they were themselves in the therapy session. The supervisor and group members may synchronise with the supervisee and may feel corresponding thoughts, emotions, and physical sensations. They may be automatically drawn to react in a certain way to repeat the dynamics of the psychotherapy relationship. The supervisor may either enact the role of the client or the role of the therapist, depending on the role the supervisee enacts. In this way, enactments in supervision may occur that are parallel to what is happening in the primary psychotherapeutic relationship.

For example, in the case of Peter, the supervisor was too compliant in supervision and did not confront Peter regarding his inability to set boundaries. He experienced Peter as strong and controlling. This pattern matched the pattern in psychotherapy, where Peter was submissive in relation to his client and experienced him as too powerful. In this case, the supervisor was repeating the therapist's role and Peter the role of his client.

In our experience, the significant dimension of the parallel process is the body/physiological dimension. Searles (1955), almost 70 years ago, described how the foundation of the parallel process is an unconscious identification with the client. Building on this, we propose that the significant component of the parallel process is the physiological synchronisation between the therapist and the client. During the psychotherapy session, the therapist's physiology tends to synchronise with the client (Bar-Kalifa et al., 2019; Messina et al., 2013; Palmieri et al., 2018; Tschacher & Meier, 2019). The therapist may experience physiological states that correspond to the clients. This is the foundation for empathy (Marci & Orr, 2006; Marci et al., 2007; Messina et al., 2013) and is linked to the quality of the therapeutic alliance (Bar-Kalifa et al., 2019; Tschacher & Meier, 2019). However, if the therapist synchronises with dysregulated physiological client's states and stays within them, this synchronisation is dysfunctional and does not lead to effective psychotherapy outcomes (G. Žvelc & Žvelc, 2021).

The supervisee's physiology in supervision parallels their physiological responses in the therapy session. For example, if the client is hyperaroused, the therapist may feel corresponding tension in their chest, faster breathing, and heartbeat. This therapist's experience is then stored in the implicit relational schema of being with the client and activated in the supervision session.

Physiological states that originate in the therapeutic relationship are then revived in the supervisory relationship. The supervisor may respond to the supervisee's physiology in the same way as the therapist did in the therapy session, for instance, not recognising the dysregulation and not initiating regulation. Alternatively, the supervisor may react differently, stop the dysfunctional synchronisation process, and initiate awareness and regulation. Mindful awareness of their physiology helps supervisors become aware of their synchronisation with their supervisees and the pattern being enacted in the supervision session.

Through awareness of their experience and their interaction with the supervisee, the supervisor may understand the dynamics of the primary psychotherapy relationship. However, the goal is not just understanding the parallel process but the transformation of both supervisor and supervisee's emotions and body sensations. Supervision is like an alchemical laboratory where transformation takes place. When enactment occurs, the physiology of both supervisor and supervisee is often dysregulated. The supervisor is mindfully aware of their own experience and the enacted interactional pattern. With the help of mindfulness and compassion interventions, the supervisor first regulates themselves and then helps to regulate the supervisee's physiology. The supervisor collaboratively with the supervisee uncovers the interactional pattern that is being enacted and forms a new relationship with the supervisee. The new relationship is contrary to the dysfunctional pattern and acts like a "mismatch" experience that is essential for memory reconsolidation of the implicit relational schema. The transformed relational schema of being with the client then positively influences the therapist's subsequent therapy sessions.

In supervision with Peter, the supervisor recognised his own internal experience (countertransference), which was manifested in compliance, feelings of fear, and tension in the chest. By bringing mindful awareness to himself, he started to decentre from his synchronisation with the supervisee and started to calm down. Regaining his inner space helped him regulate the supervisee's physiology. He invited Peter to the mindful awareness of his body sensations and helped him to get in touch with his fear of the client. Through mindful processing of the fear, Peter's way of being transformed into a sense of strength and security. The supervisor also openly addressed the issue of boundaries in supervision and therapy sessions. After supervision, Peter's way of being was changed – he experienced more strength and felt able to act in the best interest of the client. The new interactional pattern, manifested in a safe and balanced relationship in supervision, was then taken back to psychotherapy.

Chapter 4

Emotional and physiological regulation as the fourth supervision function

This chapter emphasises emotional and physiological regulation as crucial supervision processes. In our research (M. Žvelc 2015, 2017), we noticed that therapists often came from therapy sessions to supervision sessions upset and agitated. During their supervision session, if it was effective, they calmed down and became grounded and present. We found that emotional regulation was vital to the supervision process.

Even though emotional regulation is recognised as a crucial process in psychotherapy (Hill, 2015; Ogden et al., 2006; Rothschild, 2017; G. Žvelc & Žvelc, 2021), its application to supervision is barely mentioned in the literature. In this chapter, we introduce the significance of emotional and physiological regulation in the supervision process based on our own research (M. Žvelc, 2015, 2017), intersubjective physiology research (Palumbo et al., 2017), the concept of window of tolerance (D. J. Siegel, 1999, 2012), and clinical practice. Because of its importance, we call it the fourth supervision function (M. Žvelc, 2015) alongside the three well-known developmental, resourcing, and qualitative functions (Hawkins & Shohet, 2012).

Emotional and physiological regulation in supervision

Emotional regulation is the ability of an individual to tolerate and modulate their emotional state to adaptively meet the demands of their environment (Fonagy et al., 2004). It has three dimensions: Capacity to tolerate affect, modulate affect intensity, and affective resilience (Hill, 2015). Affective resilience is the capacity of a person to return efficiently to a regulated state after exposure to dysregulation. Such regulation enables integration of the mind, whereas dysregulation causes dissociation of the mind (Hill, 2015).

Our research (M. Žvelc, 2015, 2017) shows that emotional regulation is a significant process in supervision. Below we set out different forms of regulatory processes in supervision found in research. We also include a quote from a study that presents the supervisee's statement of their most significant moment in a particular supervision session. Emotional regulation processes help supervisees to move:

DOI: 10.4324/9781003194118-6

- From subjective feelings of hyperarousal and intensiveness of emotions towards calming down.

"When I think about the couple, I feel less uncomfortable and stressed when I think about our next session. My feelings towards them/the therapy are not so heavy anymore".

- From non-tolerable emotions towards tolerating and changing those emotions.

"I felt angry at myself and the client. During the supervision, I accepted that, calmed down, and felt connected with the client again. My feeling of competence to work with him also improved".

- From emotional withdrawal and avoidance towards experiencing and owning emotions.

"My supervisor pointed out mourning for the daughter's death, and I felt that this is not possible for the parents yet. At the same time, I realised that for me it is also very difficult to get in touch with sadness and loss and that I avoid these feelings".

- From self-doubt and self-criticism to self-confidence.

"The supervisor gave me the feedback that I used good interventions. I was touched and happy. A burden fell from my shoulders, because I was recently very doubtful of myself and my work. After supervision, I felt more competent".

All four categories are marked by the supervisee's overwhelming states (high arousal, non-tolerable emotions, self-criticism) or numbing states (not feeling emotions when they would be expected). These states are outside of the window of tolerance (D. J. Siegel, 1999, 2012). Through the supervision process, when both emotional and physiological regulation occur, the individual's physiology and emotion become regulated, and self-esteem and self-competency are re-established. Supervisees during supervision are enabled to move from not feeling safe to feeling safer. Supervision helps them to return to the window of tolerance.

The literature emphasises emotional and physiological regulation as significant variables in psychotherapeutic treatment (Dana, 2018; S. M. Geller, 2018; S. M. Geller & Porges, 2014; Hill, 2015; Levine, 2018; Ogden, 2018; Ogden et al., 2006; Rothschild, 2017; Siegel, 1999, 2012; G. Žvelc & Žvelc, 2021). Emotional and physiological dysregulation in psychotherapists leads to inappropriate emotional responses and interventions, and sometimes even to harmful behaviour (Ogden, 2018; Ogden et al., 2006; Rothschild, 2017;

G. Žvelc & Žvelc, 2021). Dysregulated states of the therapist are also con-nected to burnout (Rothschild, 2006) and autonomic dysregulation syndrome (Levine, 2018).

However, applying emotional regulation to supervision is rare in literature and has not yet been sufficiently researched. Bennett (2008) theoretically discusses the meaning of affect regulation in supervision related to attach-ment styles. She also presents the case where supervision helped the super-visee regulate the anxiety stimulated by her countertransference. With the help of emotional regulation, the supervisee felt less frightened by her client, which enabled her to become disembedded from the relational matrix. Champe et al. (2013) theoretically apply Gross's (2001) process model of emotion regulation in group work training and supervision. Rožič (2018), in an empirical study, found that affect regulation occurs at the pivotal moments of supervision, which are connected to the repair of disconnections in the supervisory relationship. When affect regulation takes place, the members of the supervision reconnect, feel calm and safe, and perceive themselves and their further work with their clients differently. They also gain new insights (Rožič, 2018).

Emotional and physiological regulation are interwoven and closely con-nected. Each emotion has a physiological component, and if we want to regulate the emotion, we have to regulate the physiology. When we talk about regulation, we have in mind both emotional and physiological regulation. Because of its interconnectedness and the primacy of physiological regula-tion, and because sometimes a person experiences sensations that cannot be categorised as an emotion but are nevertheless significant for the supervision process, we use the term physiological regulation more often in this chapter and throughout the book.

Our view of physiological regulation is that it is "a process of modulating the physiological arousal states of a person, bringing them to an optimal arousal zone" (G. Žvelc & Žvelc, 2021, p. 69). In the process of physiological regulation, we want to bring the defensive physiological states into balance between the sympathetic and parasympathetic branches of the nervous system, at the level of the social engagement system (Porges, 2017). In supervision, this would mean that if either member of supervision (supervisee or supervisor) is in hyperarousal, then down-regulation is needed, lowering the activation of the autonomic nervous system (ANS) and bringing it to the optimal level. If the supervisee's or supervisor's physiology is hypoaroused, their ANS's activation should be heightened. For better understanding, let us explain the main categories of physiological states.

Physiological states

We use the words physiological states and states of ANS interchangeably. Authors categorise physiological states in various ways. For clinical application to supervision, we classify physiological states on three primary levels, based on the concept of the window of tolerance (Ogden et al., 2006; D. J. Siegel, 1999, 2012) and the polyvagal theory (Porges, 2017): Optimal physiological arousal, hyperarousal, and hypoarousal. Optimal arousal is connected to feeling safe with regulated physiology, while hyperarousal and hypoarousal states are usually connected to feeling unsafe and present dysregulated physiology. According to polyvagal theory, these various states are led by the ventral vagus, sympathetic pathways, and dorsal vagus (Porges, 2011). The ventral and dorsal vagus are branches of the parasympathetic nervous system (Porges, 2017). We could describe the sympathetic and parasympathetic components of ANS as the accelerator and the brakes of the processes in the organism.

The polyvagal theory proposes the phylogenetically ordered hierarchy of the states, in which the phylogenetically newer circuits react first. They respond in the following order: Ventral vagus, sympathetic nervous system, and dorsal vagus (Porges, 2017). The nervous system continuously automatically, without our awareness, scans the internal or external environment and evaluates if it is safe, dangerous, or if there is a life threat. Porges (2017) calls this process *neuroception*. Feeling safe is connected to the ventral vagus and social engagement. When we evaluate a threat, the sympathetic branch activates first, and if we assess that fight or flight will not be sufficient, we slide to immobilisation with the help of the dorsal vagus.

Optimal arousal and window of tolerance

Optimal arousal of ANS is indicated by the balance between the sympathetic and parasympathetic branches (Hill, 2015; Murison, 2016). According to Porges (2017), the activation of the ventral vagus plays a vital role in this state. The optimal arousal zone is connected to a feeling of being safe. In the optimal arousal zone, we can feel and tolerate our emotions and sensations, and our self-regulation, resilience, and cognitive processes, including reflection, are optimal (Hill, 2015; Levine, 2018; Ogden et al., 2006). We are socially engaged in functional ways and open to learning. D. J. Siegel (1999, 2012) named this optimal zone the window of tolerance because, within it, we can tolerate present emotions and accompanying physiological processes. The width of the window represents the capacity for tolerating the affect; the wider it is, the more affect we can handle without becoming dysregulated. This means that the window of tolerance also includes some levels of hyper- or hypo-arousal of ANS, which we can tolerate (for instance, being angry and acting self-assertively instead of acting out). During this moderate arousal, our left brain and secondary process are dominant (Hill, 2015).

The window of tolerance is the optimal physiological and mental state for supervision work. In the supervision process, we strive that all parties would be or would arrive in this state of mind. We suggest that the supervisee is open to learning in this state and that their emotional and cognitive capacities, including reflection, are optimal. The same applies to the supervisor, who will more effectively lead the supervision in the optimal arousal state.

Hyperarousal

The hyperarousal of ANS is led by the sympathetic nervous system and is connected to mobilised defensive fight or flight behaviour (Ogden et al., 2006; Porges, 2011). When someone is in danger, their body uses its resources for defence, either for fighting or running away. Heart rate and blood pressure increase, and energy is channelled to the musculature (Murison, 2016). The sympathetic nervous system influences the cardiovascular system, the gastro-intestinal tract, respiration, renal, endocrine, and other systems (Murison, 2016). In supervision, this can be seen in the following ways: The supervisee talks fast or loudly, breathes rapidly or does not have time to take a breath, is restless, emotionally reactive, and hyper-vigilant, as if on guard. Their cognitive pro-cesses are not well organised; they can be confused and have difficulty hearing and using the supervisor's feedback. Introspectively, they feel too many sen-sations or disturbing emotions (Ogden et al., 2006). The supervisor may phys-iologically synchronise with a supervisee and also feel in their body restlessness, pounding of heartbeat, perspiring, etc. In these physiological states and corre-sponding states of mind, the feeling of safety is lacking. The person is not open or suitable for functional social interactions, neither for reflecting nor learning.

Therapists with preoccupied attachment styles are more prone to become hyperaroused in the therapy session (Hill, 2015). They tend to merge with clients, do not keep enough emotional distance, and can be caught by dys-regulated countertransference reactions. This often leads them to exhaustion and, for some, to burnout. We would also suggest that supervisees with preoccupied attachment styles tend to become hyperaroused in the supervi-sion session more often or more quickly.

In mild hyperarousal, we are active and alert (Rothschild, 2017). If this state is coupled with the ventral vagus circuit and the social engagement system, we feel safe enough (Porges, 2017), and we function within the window of tolerance.

Hypoarousal

Hypoarousal of ANS can vary from lethargic states (apathy, lack of energy, slow heart rate, and shallow respiration) (Rothschild, 2017) to freezing and collapsing (Ogden et al., 2006; Porges, 2017). The state is connected to immobilisation behaviour and, according to Porges (2017), is led by the dorsal vagus, a branch of the parasympathetic system. It is activated when a person senses a threat and begins to feel terror and automatically concludes that the fight/flight response is not or will not be effective. When this occurs, an animal or a person uses freezing, collapsing, dissociation, and shutting down. For instance, this state can often be seen in a mouse feigning death in front of a cat. Predators usually won't be interested in catching and eating a corpse. By analogy to the example of the mouse, a person can, on a psychological and behavioural level, feel or act "dead". If, in hyperarousal, a person feels too much and is overwhelmed, in hypoarousal, they feel too little or almost nothing.

This state can be observed during supervision by reduced body movement or stillness, paleness of skin, lowering the voice and eye gaze, inactivity, numbing of emotions, and disruptive cognitive processing. A supervisee may not feel sensations and emotions, or they can feel some unpleasant feelings in the area below the diaphragm (for instance, in the belly). A supervisor may physiologically synchronise with a supervisee and feel freezing coldness or tingling in their limbs, difficulty in breathing, inability to make a move, abdominal pain, etc. The immobilised state represents even greater danger and lack of security than the mobilised state, with the ability for social engagement being significantly reduced, as well as the ability to reflect and learn.

Therapists with avoidant attachment styles tend to enter hypoarousal more frequently than therapists with other attachment styles (secure, preoccupied) (Hill, 2015). When facing an intensive emotional display by their clients, avoidant therapists tend to close themselves emotionally and withdraw. We suggest that supervisees with avoidant attachment styles also tend to become physiologically hypoaroused and emotionally less available in the supervision session.

If the state is coupled with activation of the ventral vagus circuit, then it can lead to intimacy, deep relaxation, and meditative states (Dana, 2018; Porges, 2017).

Identification of physiological states in supervision

For effective supervision, the involved parties must be aware of their physiological states. Awareness of dysregulated physiological states helps the supervisee and supervisor to start regulating and then reflecting on the meaning of their dysregulation. We suggest that a supervisor should introduce the supervisee as early as possible to the significance of physiological states in the supervision practice. It is helpful to make a contract with supervisees in terms like: "*In supervision, we will raise awareness of the body processes and evaluate our physiological states*". The scale of physiological arousal (Žvelc & Žvelc, 2021) is a concrete tool we can use in supervision to evaluate both our and our supervisees' arousal and physiological states. We introduce supervisees to the scale (see Figure 4.1). During supervision sessions, we ask the supervisee, especially when we notice their arousal is increasing or decreasing, to evaluate their physiological arousal on the physiological scale from −5 to 5. The left side of the scale, spreading from −5 to −1, presents different levels of hypoarousal; −5 means the most intensive hypoarousal. Hypoarousal refers to feeling numb, frozen, having

How would you assess your arousal on a scale from -5 to +5?
- 5 is the most frozen or collapsed you have ever felt,
0 is optimal arousal,
and +5 is the most upset and disturbed you have ever felt in your life.

Hypoarousal   -5 -4 -3 -2 -1 **0** 1 2 3 4 5   **Hyperarousal**

Feeling numb	Feeling calm	Feeling upset
Collapsed	Relaxed	Feeling disturbed
Feeling frozen	Feeling safe	Feeling anxious
"Empty-headed"	Focused	Nervous
Spacing out	Grounded	Heart beating

Figure 4.1 Scale of physiological arousal.

Note: Reprinted from *Integrative psychotherapy: A mindfulness- and compassion-oriented approach* (p. 190), by G. Žvelc & M. Žvelc, 2021, Routledge. Copyright 2021 by Routledge. Reprinted with permission of the publisher (Taylor & Francis Ltd, www.tandfonline.com).

difficulties feeling the body, empty-headed, or spacing out. The right side of the scale represents hyperarousal, spreading from 1 to 5; 5 means the most intensive hyperarousal the person has ever felt. Hyperarousal shows in being upset, agitated, anxious, or nervous; heartbeat and breathing are fast. Number 0 represents the optimal arousal state, the equilibrium, where a person feels grounded, focused, and safe.

Physiological regulation during a supervision session

Figure 4.2 shows the course of the physiological regulation process during the supervision session. Supervisees may, during the supervision session, become emotionally and physiologically dysregulated. The supervisee may come to the session already dysregulated or become dysregulated when discussing a particular therapy case. If the supervisee experiences hyperarousal, the supervisor helps them to downregulate their physiology and differentiate the emotion. If the supervisee is in hypoarousal, we focus on raising the level of physiological arousal and leading the supervisee to come back into contact with their body and emotions. During an effective supervision session, these states become regulated, and the supervisee returns to the window of tolerance (see Figure 4.2). When entering the next therapy session, the supervisee will hopefully start and lead the therapy session from the optimal arousal zone and regulated affect.

The significance of emotional and physiological regulation in supervision

Can supervision be effective if the members of the supervision have dysregulated emotional or physiological states? We propose that dysregulated

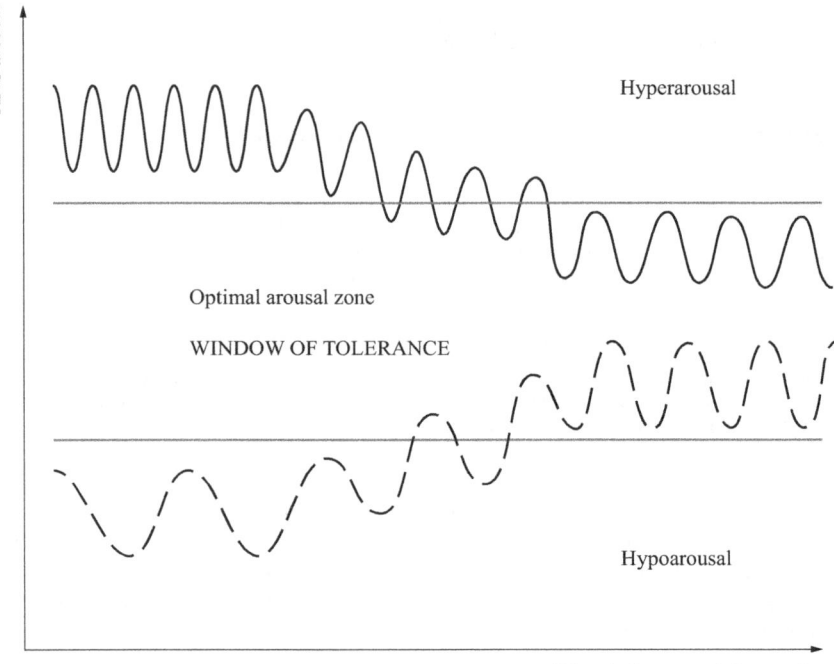

Figure 4.2 Physiological regulation throughout a supervision session.

Note: Adapted from "Sensorimotor psychotherapy: One method for processing traumatic memory" by P. Ogden, & K. Minton, 2000, *Traumatology, 6*(3) p. 158 (https://doi.org/10.1177/1534765 60000600302). Copyright 2000 by American Psychological Association- Journals. Adapted with permission of the publisher (American Psychological Association- Journals).

emotional and physiological states paralyse the supervision process and also hinder the efficiency of psychotherapy.

Hyper- and hypo-arousal states, if they are not within the window of tolerance, are defensive systems where we feel a threat, and our attention and energy are directed to attack or protect. Physiology and emotions are dysregulated in these states, and the mind is dissociated. At this level of arousal, the right, holistic, non-conscious, nonverbal primary processing prevails (Hill, 2015). Supervision in either of these two states is less or even noneffective (M. Žvelc, 2017) because reflection and mentalisation, which are pivotal for the supervision process, are compromised. The openness to learning and the range of information that can be processed are limited. The members of supervision may misinterpret the comments, suggestions, questions, and emotions of other supervision members. Their psychological flexibility (S. C. Hayes et al., 2012) is limited. Supervisees in these states cannot reflect and process their countertransference. Countertransference, which is not reflected and processed, compromises further psychotherapeutic work and can lead to unethical conduct, emotional exhaustion, and burnout. Also, if dysregulated, the supervisor cannot lead the supervision optimally and is vulnerable to burnout. We propose that therapists and supervisors would make less ethical mistakes if they could effectively recognise dysregulated emotions and physiology, regulate them, and find the meaning of their processes.

In supervision, we want to help the therapist regain regulated, balanced physiology and a secure, positive sense of self and competence.

The essential premises of mindfulness- and compassion-oriented integrative supervision is that the supervision session is effective if:

1 The members of supervision are mindfully aware of their physiological and emotional states.
2 The supervision system, involving both supervisor and supervisees, is regulated. A regulated supervision system means that the supervisor and the supervisee (or supervisees if there is group supervision) are in their social engagement system within the window of tolerance.
3 There are successful attempts at emotional and physiological regulation during the supervision session.
4 The meaning of dysregulated states is explored.

We accordingly emphasise that the crucial process in supervision is that dysregulated states of supervisees and supervisors are recognised, returned to optimal states of arousal, and understood and mentalised. To achieve this, the supervisor should be in an optimal arousal state, or they should recognise when they are approaching or crossing the edges of the window of tolerance and start to regulate themselves. The fundamental task of the supervisor is to track the supervisees' and their own physiological states to help the supervisee be aware of their physiological and emotional states during supervision sessions (and during therapy), assisting supervisees in regulating the states and understanding the meaning of them. Because of its high significance, we propose emotional and physiological regulation as the fourth function of the supervision process alongside the three well-known developmental, resourcing, and qualitative functions (Hawkins & Shohet, 2012).

When the emotions and physiology of supervision members are regulated, they can efficiently adapt to the requirements of supervision and utilise their resources; they can explore, reflect, and mentalise about their states and their clients' internal state and are open to learning. Awareness of the body and its physiological states also helps the supervisor and supervisee to stay present during the supervision session. They are able to think and feel. So we can say when the members of the supervision are regulated, they function optimally. Supervision is the place where we want the supervisee to learn and grow, and this is possible only within regulated physiology and emotions. The regulation of physiology and emotions helps the supervision members to be emotionally more stable in their psychotherapy practice. With this, we also prevent the emotional distress and burnout of professionals.

By regulating the supervisee's physiology and emotions, we are giving the therapist the resources to provide secure experiences and effective interventions to their clients through the reverse parallel process. Based on our clinical supervision practice, we can justly say that by regulation in supervision, we are not just improving supervision outcomes but therapy outcomes as well.

To understand the interaction of dysregulated states among members of psychotherapy and supervision and effectively regulate ourselves, it is essential to understand the processes of intersubjective physiology and physiological synchrony.

Intersubjective physiology and physiological synchrony in supervision

Intersubjective theory emphasises that each phenomenon in the individual should be considered within a wider intersubjective, relational context (Stolorow, 1994). There is a mutual influence among interacting people. A significant part of this mutual influence flows nonverbally between our bodies. The changes in physiology of one person should thus be viewed within a wider context. This means that interaction with other people influences the physiology of an individual. The concept of intersubjective physiology includes the reciprocal influencing processes, which occur between the interconnected physiologies of two or more people (G. Žvelc & Žvelc, 2021). This is confirmed by research showing that social processes among people also flow at an implicit, physiological level (for review, see Palumbo et al., 2017). The nervous systems of two or more people interact (Palumbo et al., 2017; Porges, 2011, 2017; Schore, 2019). The concept of intersubjective physiology is connected to concepts such as emotional contagion (Hatfield et al., 2014), emotional resonance (D. J. Siegel, 2007), automatic mimicry (Prochazkova & Kret, 2017), and mirror neurons (di Pellegrino et al., 1992; Ferrari & Gallese, 2007).

Intersubjective physiology is being researched and proved through measurements of physiological synchrony, which illustrate the connectedness between the physiological activities of two or more people. Physiological synchrony studies have measured physiological processes (such as the frequency of the heartbeat, heart rate variability, respiration activity, skin conduction, cortisol levels, etc.) among mother–child dyads, family members, partners, group members, and psychotherapist–client dyads. The studies show that the participants' physiology tends to synchronise (Bar-Kalifa et al., 2019; Karvonen et al., 2016; Päivinen et al., 2016; Palmieri et al., 2018; Palumbo et al., 2017; Saxbe & Repetti, 2010; Saxbe et al., 2014; Suveg et al., 2016; Tschacher & Meier, 2019). For instance, Saxbe et al. (2014) examined the association of cortisol levels of 103 family triads and found that the cortisol levels of mothers, fathers, and adolescents were positively correlated. They also found specific patterns of physiological influence between family members: The mother's cortisol levels predicted the father's cortisol levels, the father's predicted the youth's, and the youth's cortisol levels predicted the mother's.

Different studies of physiological synchrony in individual or couple therapy show a correlation in heart rate, heart rate variability, electrodermal activity, skin conductance, and respiration between therapists and their clients (Bar-Kalifa et al., 2019; Karvonen et al., 2016; Päivinen et al., 2016; Palmieri et al., 2018; Tschacher & Meier, 2019). Sympathetic and parasympathetic connectedness were also found in therapy dyads (Tschacher & Meier, 2019). Research has shown connections between physiological synchrony and a good therapeutic alliance (Bar-Kalifa et al., 2019; Tschacher & Meier, 2019) and the therapist's empathy (Marci & Orr, 2006; Marci et al., 2007; Messina et al., 2013; Robinson et al., 1982).

In the overview of physiological synchrony research in psychotherapy, Kleinbub et al. (2020) note that there is an increasing number but still only a small number of research studies. They conclude that psychotherapy practice can benefit greatly from this kind of research. We agree with them and would like to add that this is also true for supervision. We have not found any study of physiological synchrony in psychotherapy supervision. We suggest that the supervision field would be enriched by research on the physiological processes of supervision members.

We also consider that research on two types of physiological synchrony is needed, functional and dysfunctional. We suggest that the studies mentioned above, which show a connection between physiological synchrony and good therapeutic alliance, relate to functional synchrony. Practitioners and researchers should also pay attention to dysfunctional synchrony, which needs to be examined.

In the following subchapter, we present these two types of physiological synchrony and their role in clinical practice.

Functional and dysfunctional physiological synchrony

We divide physiological synchrony into two categories: Functional and dysfunctional. This division is crucial and very helpful for psychotherapeutic and supervision work. The division is based on our clinical findings and Helm's et al. (2014) categorisation on *morphostatic* and *morphogenic* synchrony, studied within romantic couples. The first kind of synchrony leads to regulation and is connected to relationship satisfaction. The second leads to dysregulation and is related to relationship dissatisfaction and conflicts (Helm et al., 2014).

Physiological synchrony is functional when it occurs in the optimal physiological arousal zone (or near it). It provides physiological regulation of the persons involved. It enables a psychotherapist or supervisor to feel the other person's feelings and respond appropriately. In other words, it allows attunement and compassion. In this kind of synchrony, involved parties, even though connected, are not merged. They sustain the optimal distance between them and keep a decentred perspective towards their inner states. Reflection and mentalisation are available. Functional synchronisation leads to feelings of connectedness and understanding. It is pervaded with a feeling of being safe.

Dysfunctional physiological synchrony happens when two or more persons synchronise in dysregulated physiological states. If the psychotherapist and the client, or supervisor and supervisee, are in hyperarousal or hypoarousal, then their physiological synchronisation is dysfunctional. In this kind of synchronisation, boundaries between people have blurred, and reflection and mentalisation are limited. Synchronising with the dysfunctional state of the other often leads to a downward spiral, with the physiology of both parties becoming increasingly dysregulated. This means that psychotherapy or supervision members get increasingly anxious, upset, or closed and numb. It is essential that therapists recognise the signs of dysfunctional synchrony, interrupt it, regulate themselves, and then lead the client to synchronise with their regulated state (G. Žvelc & Žvelc, 2021). If not recognised and further prevented, we suggest dysfunctional physiological synchrony may lead to poor psychotherapy, therapist's emphatic distress, and burnout (G. Žvelc & Žvelc, 2021). The same is valid for supervision.

Clinical application of the intersubjective physiology concept

Based on the research and our own clinical findings, we emphasise that the physiological states of the therapist and the client are interconnected and tend to synchronise. The therapist responds to the client's physiology and the client to the therapist's. Because of this, we propound that the essential psychotherapeutic factor is the physiological state of the therapist during the therapy session (G. Žvelc & Žvelc, 2021). The process of functional physiological synchrony enables the therapist to sense the client's physiological states and co-regulate them. Continued mindful awareness of their own state and the clients' during the therapy session helps the therapist to interrupt dysfunctional regulation and take the lead towards self-regulation and regulation of the client. Research and clinical practice show that mindful awareness enables regulation (Farb et al., 2012; Goldin & Gross, 2010; Hayes & Feldman, 2004; Price & Hooven, 2018; Taren et al., 2013; Teper et al., 2013; Vago & Silbersweig, 2012; G. Žvelc & Žvelc, 2021).

These implicit processes of nonverbal physiological communication also exist in supervision. So why not use these automatic processes in supervision and direct them in a helpful and effective way? The role of supervision is to equip the therapist with mindful awareness, knowledge of regulation, and presence in therapy, and also to help them recognise and transform their dysregulated states during the supervision sessions.

Physiological dysregulation occurring in therapy is re-enacted in supervision. It is revealed through body interaction between the supervisor and supervisees. The supervisor and the supervisee should recognise dysregulation in supervision, then step out from it and encourage regulation processes. They can step out from a dysregulated matrix with the help of the observing self, which facilitates mindful awareness processes: Present moment awareness, acceptance, and decentred perspective.

The supervisor is responsible for being aware of their own physiological processes. Changes in the heartbeat, respiration, and other body sensations might be part of the synchronisation process with the supervisee, which may come from the therapist's and client's synchronisation. Knowing the body as a supervisor is a royal road to read the unrecognised, untold story of the therapy encounter. This story can be connected to the unconscious story of the client and their relationships (as well as the therapist's and the supervisor's story). Recognising the dysfunctional physiological synchrony also enables the supervisor and the supervisees to understand how they become dysregulated and how to accomplish regulation.

Reasons for physiological dysregulation in the supervision session

Significant processes that contribute to dysregulated physiology states in supervision are:

- The physiological parallel process is related to the transmission of the physiological dysregulated states from the therapy system to supervision system.
- A supervisory alliance rupture.

Other factors that may contribute to physiological and emotional dysregulation in supervision are as follows: The supervisee's or supervisor's criticism and self-criticism, insecure attachment, unresolved trauma, and intensive life stress of the supervisee or the supervisor.

Physiological parallel process: Transmission of dysregulation from therapy to supervision

Although supervisees in supervision talk about their clients, their relationship with them, their emotional reactions, and the methods they use, this presents only a limited picture of the therapy process. Much more of the therapy process and the therapeutic relationship is revealed through the emotions and bodily/physiological states of a supervisee, supervisor, and the group members in the supervision session. When the therapist cannot tolerate their clients' and their own affect and becomes dysregulated, this dysregulation is transmitted to the supervision session and shows in the physiological processes among the members of supervision. We call this the physiological parallel process.

Research (M. Žvelc, 2015, 2017) and our own clinical supervision practice have shown us that during a therapy session, therapists do not always recognise that the therapy system (the client, the therapist, and the space between them) is dysregulated. Because of the lack of mindful awareness of their and their clients' physiological states, therapists may miss the signs of dysregulated states. Because of the processes of physiological synchrony (Palumbo et al., 2017; G. Žvelc & Žvelc, 2021) and neuroception (Porges, 2017), unrecognised dysregulated client states implicitly influence the therapist's ANS, which becomes dysregulated too. The same is equally true the other way around. It sometimes also happens that the therapist may recognise the dysregulated therapy system but is unable to regulate it, and despite their attempts, they can neither regulate themselves nor the client.

As we explain in Chapter 3, the therapist's physiological and emotional states activated during therapy sessions are stored in the psychotherapist's implicit memory and form relational schemas of being with the client. These implicit memories related to relational schemas are triggered in the supervision session. The activation of the therapist's relational schema of being with the client is revealed in the supervisee's physiological processes (accelerated heartbeat, pressure in the chest, tingling sensations, numbing, aches in parts of the body, etc.), emotions, cognitions, and behaviour.

In this way, the supervisee transfers dysregulated physiological states from the therapy system to the supervision system. The therapist's implicit body memory, stored in the relational schema of being with the client, is a mediator from the therapeutic to the supervisory relationship. The therapist brings their dysregulated physiological countertransference, which originates in the therapeutic relationship, into the supervisory relationship. This is the physiological parallel process. Let us suppose a therapy system (a client and therapist and the space between them) is dysregulated at the end of the session. In that case, the therapist holds this dysregulated physiological state in their body. Although they may be unaware of this, they may suffer symptoms such as anxiety or agitation, accelerated or irregular heartbeat, heavy breathing, fatigue, pain in the body, sleep disturbances, digestive problems, vomiting, etc. When they come to supervision and start discussing the therapy with a particular client, their body "remembers" and starts showing the "untold, implicit story" of the therapeutic interaction. If we as supervisors want to see and understand what is going on in psychotherapy sessions, we need to listen to our and our supervisees' bodies, because the interaction of our bodies most likely parallels the interaction between the therapist's and client's bodies.

There are different interplays of therapy dysregulation, which can be transferred to supervision. They are connected to the attachment styles of the

therapist and the client (Hill, 2015). With a preoccupied client, the therapeutic dyad may quickly become hyperaroused, and with an avoiding client,
the therapeutic dyad can become hypoaroused (Hill, 2015). It is also possible
that a preoccupied therapist may be unable to tolerate the client's hypoarousal and may become hyperaroused and intrusive. In contrast, an avoidant
therapist, frightened by and unable to tolerate hyperarousal, may withdraw
and become hypoaroused (Hill, 2015). The therapist brings their hyper- or
hypo-arousal into the supervision session, and the supervisor reacts to it
according to their attachment styles.

Rupture in the supervisory alliance and other reasons for physiological dysregulation

Research shows (M. Žvelc, 2017) that dysregulated states in supervision are
not necessarily the consequence of the parallel process. There can be other
causes for it. Often it is a rupture in the supervisory alliance, and it manifests
through physiological hyper- or hypo-arousal of the supervisee and the
supervisor (and the group members if there is group supervision). In this case,
we regulate the supervision system with the help of work on rupture repair
(see Chapter 5).

The other main reason which leads to dysregulation is the high self-
criticism of the supervisee or supervisor. In this case, we use self-compassion
strategies (see Chapters 10 and 11). If a supervisee is under considerable life
stress, we are compassionate to them and discuss how this might influence the
work with their clients and what they need. If needed, we advise them to take
a self-care break or direct them to personal psychotherapy. If we as supervisors are under life stress that shows in chronic dysregulation of our ANS, it
is important to go to supervision or consultation with a senior colleague. The
adverse effects on supervision sessions by the temporary stress of the supervisee or the supervisor can be reduced by mindful preparation for the
supervision sessions and by inviting the members at the beginning of the
supervision session to acknowledge the suffering they are going through.
In that way, they reduce their emotional burden and are ready for further
supervision work. More extreme insecure attachment styles (Watkins, 1995)
and unresolved trauma of the members of supervision are hindering factors in
supervision; we think that in this case more personal therapy is needed.

Transmission of regulated physiological states from supervision to therapy

Hopefully, the supervisee, who accomplishes physiological and emotional
regulation during supervision, takes this regulated state into their psychotherapy practice. By regulation in supervision, we influence the healing
processes in the following therapy sessions.

Shaping the therapist's "way of being" and transforming their relational schemas

We, as supervisors, can influence what the supervisee will do in the following therapy session by leading them to reflect, get insights, advice, and discussion on what to do, etc. Furthermore, we can also significantly impact the supervisee's way of being: Their state of physiology and mind at the next therapy session. In our opinion, the most effective process in supervision for shaping the therapist's way of being in their work as psychotherapists is physiological regulation: Modulating the supervisee's ANS and leading it towards balance. The experiences of emotional and physiological regulation become encoded into their implicit memory. Additionally, the supervisee's dysfunctional relational schema of being with the client may transform through new experiences in their supervision, such as experiencing emotional and physiological regulation.

Supervisors help the supervisee to stay within the window of tolerance while discussing the details of psychotherapy with a particular client. The relational schemas are part of the implicit memory (D. J. Siegel, 2012). A significant part of the schema is the bodily physiological component. By regulating the supervisee's physiology while discussing the client, we may activate the process of memory reconsolidation (Ecker et al., 2012) and change the supervisee's relational schema of being with the client. This schema transformation leads to a new way of relating to the client.

Let's look at the example of the supervisee, Boris, who developed a dysfunctional schema "I feel worthless next to the client", and "I am not safe with this client". The bodily part of this relational schema was that Boris was hypoaroused in the therapy and supervision session, feeling "nothing" and immobilised regarding what to do in therapy. Through mindful awareness in supervision, Boris realised he was holding his breath. When inhaling deeply and exhaling more slowly, he got in touch with his fear and shame. The supervisor supported him in tolerating and accepting these feelings by explaining that they are common in our work and reminding Boris to breathe. Through regulation in supervision, his experience was transformed into "I am OK" and "I am safe" and, on the physiological level, into optimal arousal. This experience was juxtaposed with previous experiences of a lack of self-worth and feeling unsafe, which promoted the transformation of his dysfunctional relational schema. Because Boris' relational schema of being with the client was transformed, Boris came to the following therapy changed. His way of being with the client was different. The client noticed the change in her therapist immediately at the beginning of the session. She described Boris as being more warm and relaxed (before she experienced him as cold and critical). In therapy, Boris activated his safe physiological state, which he had gained in the supervision session. Even at the start of the therapy session, he greeted the client differently; his look, voice, facial expression, and gestures conveyed safety. We can say that a new kind of relationship was created between the therapist and the client. The client detected the cues for safety, her ANS calmed, and she used her energy to utilise therapy for her growth instead of protecting herself.

Emotional and physiological regulation during supervision sessions brings therapists to an optimal state of "body-mind" for psychotherapy. It impacts the therapists' way of being in therapy. It influences how *we are in therapy*, our quality of presence. Therapeutic presence is a way of being with clients that optimise the *doing* of the therapy (S. M. Geller & Greenberg, 2012; G. Žvelc & Žvelc, 2021). Mindful presence is one of the essential qualities of effective psychotherapy (Erskine, 2015; S. M. Geller, 2018; S. M. Geller & Greenberg, 2012; G. Žvelc & Žvelc, 2021). The regulation experienced in supervision can influence and heighten the chances that the therapist will be mindfully present during their psychotherapy work. We can also help therapists prevent burnout and other stress-related syndromes.

In this chapter, we have provided a theoretical foundation for emotional and physiological regulation in supervision. In Chapter 9, we present methods of emotional and physiological regulation in supervision through two vignettes from supervision practice.

Chapter 5

Supervisory alliance and supervisory alliance rupture repair

The supervisory working alliance refers to a collaborative bond between the supervisor and supervisee(s) with an agreement to work together towards set supervision goals (Bordin, 1983). As the word alliance suggests, the supervisor and supervisee become allies in the supervision process to encourage the supervisee's professional learning and development, enhance the quality of their therapeutic practice, and fulfil specific supervision session contracted goals. According to Bordin (1983), a supervisory alliance consists of three interrelated components: 1) Mutual agreement of supervision goals, 2) mutual agreement of supervision tasks, and 3) a bond between supervisor and supervisee(s). The first two components, the mutual agreement of supervision goals and tasks, can be described as technical components. The bond refers to the quality of the supervisory relationship and can be viewed as the relational component. All components, technical and relational, mutually influence one another (Safran & Muran, 2000). We would say that the alliance includes the quality of "feeling" of one another in the supervisory relationship and the conscious decision and intention to actively attend supervision for professional development and for providing a high-quality psychotherapy practice. The implicit feelings and explicit purposes, together with the mutual agreement on what we will do in the supervision and towards which goals, all influence the quality of the supervisory alliance.

The supervisory working alliance is an essential supervisory integrative and facilitative variable (Watkins, 2014; M. Žvelc, 2017). In the integrative model of processes of change in integrative supervision, maintaining and repairing the supervisory alliance is the core process related to the interpersonal dimension (see Table 1.1, Chapter 1). Meta-analysis of supervisory alliance research shows that the supervisory working alliance is positively related to supervision outcome (Park et al., 2019). The supervisory alliance positively correlates with supervision satisfaction, self-efficacy, self-disclosure, and working alliance in counselling (Park et al., 2019). The relationship between supervisor and supervisees strongly influences everything that happens in the supervision and indirectly influences the therapeutic process. In their meta-analysis, Park et al. (2019) found that the

DOI: 10.4324/9781003194118-7

supervisees' perceived relationship with the supervisor is related to their relationship with the client.

Contracting in supervision

The first two components of the supervisory alliance, mutual agreement of supervision goals and tasks, are related to the process of forming supervisory contracts. The third component, the bond between the supervisee and the supervisor, influences the quality of contracting in the supervision, and vice versa – good contracting improves the bond. There are three main categories of contracting in supervision: 1) The general supervisory contract or agreement at the outset of supervision, 2) the supervision session contract, and 3) process contracts.

The general supervisory agreement

When a supervisor begins supervision with a new supervisee, it is essential that at the outset the supervisor explains the way they work, what are the general supervision goals, what they expect from the supervisee, and what kind of tasks are required (like bringing transcripts, exploring emotional and physiological states, etc.), and discusses this with the supervisee. For example, in MCIS, we explain that an important focus of the supervision is paying attention to emotions and body sensations during supervision and we emphasise processes of mindful awareness, compassion, and self-regulation in the supervision process. Supervisors also inquire about the supervisee's expectations and beliefs, and if the supervisee is still in the early stages of their professional development, they may discuss and normalise the beginner's anxiety (Watkins, 2017b). Based on their mutual discussion, the supervisor and the supervisee make a written agreement that includes all the agreed formal aspects of supervision, such as setting supervision times, payment structure, cancellation policy, anticipated duration, confidentiality, and data protection (Thomas, 2007).

The supervision session contract

The supervisory session contract refers to the agreement of goals and tasks for a particular supervision session. The session contract is based on the supervisee's question or presented problem connected to their therapeutic work at the outset of the supervision session. The supervisory question or presenting problem reveals the supervisee's underlying need. A helpful question to the supervisee at the beginning of the session is: "What do you need from this supervision session"? The supervisor and the supervisee negotiate what they will work on in the session.

Research (M. Žvelc, 2015, 2017) shows that most often supervisees in the supervision session wish to work on how to proceed with the psychotherapeutic work with a specific client or explore and deal with their personal process, connected to their psychotherapeutic work.

Here is one example of session contracting in supervision:

Supervisee: *I am not looking forward to therapy. I'm feeling afraid.*

Supervisor: *I suggest that we mindfully observe and explore this feeling of fear today; it is an important countertransference phenomenon; it has a meaning of and for the therapy. If need be, we'll regulate it. How does that sound to you?*

Supervisee: *At first, I felt a little anxious 'cause I would rather avoid it. But when you suggested regulating it, I felt I was safe and protected here, so let's do it.*

Process contracts in supervision

We divide process contracts in supervision into relational process contracts and process contracts within the supervision session. The relational process contract focuses on the maintenance of the supervisory alliance. It refers to "an agreement to bring at the surface any issues that may be standing in the way of such an alliance" (M. C. Gilbert & Evans, 2000, p. 71). The contract encourages the supervisee to take responsibility for addressing if there is something in the supervision they missed or did not like (M. Žvelc, 2017); and also to let the supervisor know if their feedback was unclear (Watkins et al., 2022). The relational process contract is usually made at the outset of supervision.

Process contracts within the supervision session refer to contracting during supervision about the direction of the particular supervision session. Some call them mini-contracts (M. C. Gilbert & Evans, 2000). Process contracts may involve contracts about implementing a specific task or redefining a supervision goal. For example, in MCIS, we may, during the supervision session, ask the supervisee if they are willing to pause and mindfully observe their body sensations, and the supervisee agrees to do that.

The supervisory bond

The third component of the supervisory alliance, the bond, refers to the quality of the relationship between the supervisor and the supervisee or supervisees if there is group supervision. A good supervisory bond consists of feelings of trust, care, support, liking (Bordin, 1983), and safety. These feelings are at the roots of supervision; they facilitate and influence all activity in supervision. If there is no safety or trust in the supervisory relationship, the supervision work will be limited, and supervisees will more often conceal elements of their therapeutic work, feelings, and ideas (Ladany et al., 2001; Žvelc, 2017). They will avoid doing some tasks in supervision, and finally, they may leave. When there are no mutual feelings of trust, safety, and support in the supervisory relationship, there is an alliance rupture. In integrative relational supervision, we emphasise the primary importance of a good supervisory relationship and working on alliance ruptures if they happen in the supervision process (M. C. Gilbert & Evans, 2000).

The technical and relational factors of the supervisory alliance are connected and influence each other (Safran & Muran, 2000). By successfully negotiating the goals and tasks, we provide safety; with a good bond, it is easier to make supervision contracts, and the motivation to adhere to them is higher.

Research confirms that the quality of the supervisory alliance, especially the bond component, is connected to good and effective supervision (Carter et al., 2009; Henderson et al., 1999; Jacobsen & Tanggaard, 2009; Martin et al., 1987; Park et al., 2019; Rabinowitz et al., 1986; Worthen & McNeill, 1996; Worthington & Roehlke, 1979). The supervisory alliance is also linked to supervisees' satisfaction with supervision (Ladany et al., 1999) and supervisees' self-disclosure (Ladany et al., 2001; M. Žvelc & Žvelc, 2021). A poor supervision alliance is connected to conflictual situations in supervision (Gray et al., 2001; Hsu & Tsai, 2006; Nelson & Friedlander, 2001; Quarto, 2003; M. Žvelc, 2017).

The question is: How to establish a good supervisory alliance and how to maintain and repair it? The alliance is not static – it is a dynamic phenomenon. Ruptures in the alliance are inevitable (Guistolise, 1996; M. Žvelc, 2008). The quality of the alliance depends on all parties in the relationship: The supervisor and the supervisee. It is, therefore, dependent not only on the supervisor. In our research and supervision training, we found that Slovenian supervisors are too critical of themselves and place too high a responsibility on themselves (M. Žvelc, 2017).

We should ask ourselves, as supervisors, how can we promote a good supervisory alliance? There is a significant relationship between a good supervisory alliance and the supervisor's open and empathic style of supervision, as well as their humility, presence, and mindfulness (Keil, 2016; Ladany et al., 2001; Watkins, 2017b; Watkins et al., 2019; M. Žvelc, 2017).

Supervisor's attunement and mindful presence

The supervisor's ability to form healthy and secure relationships is vital for the supervisory alliance (White & Queener, 2003). The supervisor, with their style, way of being, and attitude towards the supervisees, strongly influences the quality of the supervisory alliance and, through that, impacts the efficacy of the supervision. Through their style, they are also modelling how to be in therapy. Supervisees value supervisors who are respectful, empathic, warm and attuned, open, present, and involved (M. Žvelc, 2017). An open attitude refers to the supervisor's openness towards different opinions and ideas, which the supervisee has, towards different theoretical concepts, techniques, and methods, also from other psychotherapeutic schools, and openness concerning sociocultural differences.

Other favourable characteristics of the supervisor from the supervisee's point of view are that they are sincere, accessible, knowledgeable, and skilled; they respect the contract, self-disclose, and use humour (Žvelc, 2015, 2017). Similarly, Ladany et al. (2001) confirmed that attractive (warm, supportive, and friendly) and sensitive (involved with empathic understanding) supervisory styles positively influence the supervisory alliance. Other research has also shown a positive link between supervisors' self-disclosure and the supervisory alliance (Davidson, 2011; Knox et al., 2011; Ladany & Lehrman-Waterman, 1999). The strongest connection was found between supervisors' disclosure of their difficulties in their counselling work and the bond component of the supervisory alliance (Ladany & Lehrman-Waterman, 1999). Self-disclosure of the supervisor's vulnerabilities is a powerful intervention for encouraging the supervisory relationship.

Research also supports the connection between the supervisor's mindfulness and the quality of the supervisory alliance and the supervisees' perception of self-efficacy (Keil, 2016). Mindfully based supervisors use relational inquiry, listening and pausing, encouraging mindfulness of the body, a not knowing stance, and openness towards vulnerability (Evans, 2018). More recently, the emphasis is also on the supervisor's humility (Watkins et al., 2019) which matches these described features of the supervisor.

With this described attitude of the supervisor, there is a higher chance that the supervisee will feel safe, accepted, and supported in the supervisory relationship. Safety is our primary need (Maslow, 1943). Our neurological system is constantly through the process of *neuroception* detecting if we are safe or in danger (Porges, 2017). The same is happening in supervision. If the supervisee feels safe, they will mobilise their energy towards learning and creativity, but if they do not feel safe, they will activate their defence mechanism for protection. Safety in the relationship is the basis of secure attachments. Only within a secure attachment can a child explore the world, learn, and develop optimally. The same holds true for the supervisee; only within a secure attachment to supervision can the supervisee explore their feelings, ideas, and actions freely and develop optimally professionally.

Research shows the supervisor's attachment styles significantly impact the supervisory alliance (Dickson et al., 2011; Riggs & Bretz, 2006; White & Queener, 2003). However, where some supervisees have strongly insecure attachment patterns, it is difficult or sometimes impossible to build a good bond with them (Watkins, 1995) despite the supervisor's open, empathic, and securely attached style.

Supervisees openness to learning and compassionate awareness

Supervisees are the other side of the supervisory relationship coin and are also part of creating this relationship. We must not overlook the supervisee as a significant supervisory factor (Watkins, 2017b; M. Žvelc, 2017). The features, which contribute positively to the supervisory alliance, are the supervisee's motivation and openness to learning and self-exploration, ability to self-reflect, capacity for self-acceptance, and compassionate awareness of their own and other people's vulnerabilities and strengths (Angus & Kagan, 2007; Safran et al., 2008; M. Žvelc, 2017). The attachment style of the supervisee is also related to their perception of the supervisory bond (Renfro-Michel & Sheperis, 2009).

In supervision, it is hugely important that the supervisee is intrinsically motivated for supervision and for fulfilling supervision tasks (such as preparing for the supervision session by writing transcripts, etc.). Supervisees also need to be willing to explore their inner experiences and be able to approach them with kindness and compassion, whatever they are. The supervisory relationship also benefits if the supervisee does not suffer from a severely insecure attachment style and unresolved trauma, enabling them to feel safer in the supervisory relationship. The capacity for mindful awareness, self-reflection, and self-compassion helps supervisees to decentre from their inner critic and false inferences about what the supervisor might think of them. This will help them to regulate themselves effectively, protecting themselves from internal criticism and shame. With group supervision, the secure relational schemas and attachment styles of the supervisees are also of high significance for creating and maintaining a supportive atmosphere in the supervisory group. Supervisees with insecure relational schemas are prone to experience shame within the group and may significantly disengage from the supervision process (M. Žvelc, 2017).

In the following excerpt from our research (M. Žvelc, 2017), we first hear how the supervisee shares with the researcher how she used to criticise herself with harsh and blaming words when the supervisor inquired about her psychotherapy work. Afterwards, we see how the supervisee tells the researcher that she managed to decentre from her tormented inner thoughts of criticism and was able to tolerate them. We can see she regulated herself and regained her sense of safety, ready to engage more flexibly in the supervisory relationship: "*You don't work OK! You're not OK! It is no good! When I got these thoughts, I froze. Recently, I managed to understand that the supervisor is only asking me something relevant to supervision; he is just interested in what I wanted to say. And I tell him, and the conversation goes on normally*".

Intersubjectivity and physiological regulation in the supervisory relationship

The supervisor's and supervisee's features combine uniquely in the mutual, intersubjective field of the supervisory relationship, which is embedded in the intersubjective matrix, where all sides influence each other. A significant portion of the relational processes run implicitly, beyond awareness. We are particularly interested in intersubjective physiology, the concept that describes one person's physiology influencing the physiology of the other and vice versa. In recent years, intersubjective physiology has been given more attention and research in psychotherapy (Kleinbub et al., 2020; Palmieri et al., 2021; G. Žvelc & Žvelc, 2021). In MCIS, we apply the concept of intersubjective physiology to supervision.

For the relational work of supervision, it is of the utmost importance that the supervisor and the supervisee are both mindfully aware of their experience of the supervisory relationship here and now, which Safran and Muran (2000) call "mindfulness in action". The awareness of body processes, emotions, and fantasies gives them significant information about the implicit inter-subjective field of the supervisory relationship. It may also reveal the features of the discussed psychotherapy process. In a safe supervisory relationship, the supervisor leads the supervisee towards their mindful awareness of their experiences; at the same time, the supervisor is modelling their mindful presence. Where the supervision members detect some uneasiness or conflict in the relationship, it is important to address them and meta-communicate about the processes in the relationship (Safran et al., 2008).

Mindful awareness of physiological processes helps supervisors detect physiological and emotional dysregulation. Detecting signs of hyperarousal (e.g. fast heartbeat, quick breath rhythm, sweating, restlessness in the limbs, etc.) or hypoarousal (e.g. slow heartbeat or breath rhythm, not feeling the body, coldness in the limbs, etc.) in the supervisor or the supervisee may indicate that one or very likely both of them are dysregulated.

As the quality of the mother–child relationship is indicated by their patterns of affect regulation (Schore, 1994), the quality of the supervisory alliance is related to successful emotional and physiological regulation in the supervisory relationship. The supervisor's task is to detect the dysregulation and help themselves and the supervisee to regain regulation. In that way, the supervisee goes to the following psychotherapy session transformed, with regulated emotions and physiology. The supervisee's optimal arousal implicitly and explicitly influences the therapeutic process. The supervisee may implicitly regulate their client with their own regulated emotional and physiological state. As their arousal is within the window of tolerance, their cognitive functioning is optimal, and they may make wiser and more appropriate decisions about leading the therapy. A more detailed description of this process is given in Chapters 4 and 9.

Dysregulated emotions and physiology in the supervisory relationship are related to supervisory alliance ruptures.

Supervisory alliance ruptures

Supervision ruptures refer to a "potentially problematic relational event or set of events between supervisor and supervisee" (Watkins, 2021, p. 3) or to the outcome of an unresolved supervisory impasse (Watkins, 2021), which leads to a deterioration in the quality of the supervisory relationship or even drop out (M. Žvelc, 2017). Based on Safran and Muran's (2000) model of rupture resolutions, supervision ruptures can be categorised into two types: Confrontational and withdrawal (Safran et al., 2008). In confrontational ruptures, the supervisees express their anger or dissatisfaction regarding the supervisor or supervision, whereas, in withdrawal ruptures, supervisees withdraw from the supervisory relationship or their emotional or other inner processes (Safran et al., 2008). This can show in being late for supervision, not bringing a prepared case to supervision, storytelling, or "always" agreeing. Because of the power difference in supervision, withdrawal ruptures are more common (Watkins, 2021; M. Žvelc, 2017).

When there is a good supervisory alliance, the supervision members do not pay much attention to it; it is like a steady background or solid ground on which you can build the structure. However, when something is wrong in the supervisory relationship, this becomes very figural and omits the supervisory work. In our supervision research, when the alliance was good, the supervision members did not mention much about the significance of the supervisory alliance (M. Žvelc, 2017). However, when we asked them what was hindering a session, a broken supervisory bond was present in almost every case. Safran et al. (2008) similarly suggest that the relationship does not have to be addressed explicitly when the alliance is good. When tensions emerge, then exploration of the relationship should be the priority.

Problematic relational events in the supervision session

Problematic relational events may be a sign of a rupture or may lead to the rupture of the supervisory alliance. This subchapter presents some problematic, hindering events from real supervision sessions that we encountered in our research of facilitative and hindering factors in supervision (M. Žvelc, 2017). To illustrate different categories of problematic events, we have added concrete statements from the supervision members about how they experienced the impasse.

Ruptures in the supervisory alliance showed in the form of conflicts and problems in the supervisory relationship, disagreement over goals and methods, or were related to the dual roles of supervision members. Here is what a supervisee had to say, written after one of the supervision sessions, where we detected disagreement in goals and methods (M. Žvelc, 2017): "*I see no point in dealing just with the past because it often does not change anything. My supervisor thinks that only working in the past, deep work, is the only right way to do the therapy; and I don't agree with that*". From the interview, we found out that the supervisee was very dissatisfied with the supervision and was withdrawing as much as she could from the supervisory relationship, giving a minimum of information and a minimum of herself. This was a clear sign of a supervisory rupture. The supervisor sensed the impasse in the relationship. After the same supervision session, she interestingly wrote: *"I can't deeply connect with this supervisee. I feel I should talk about my feelings that we are not on the same line. That I cannot go deeper with her. I wish so much to sense her better, but I can't. I would like to ask her how she is experiencing our relationship and what she would need from me"*.

Supervisor's characteristics contributing to alliance ruptures

In our research (M. Žvelc, 2017), we found that the following characteristics of supervisors in supervision sessions contributed to supervisory alliance ruptures: The supervisor was authoritative, not respectful, humiliating, abusing trust, and displaying irresponsible behaviour. For example, one supervisee noted the disrespectful behaviour of the supervisor towards the supervisee's clients: *"I wish she wouldn't imitate the client foolishly and that she wouldn't roll her eyes when I talk about my client"*.

In another case, the supervisor humiliated the supervisee: *"Once when we were practising, my supervisor was rude: 'What are you doing?!?? Do you have any idea?!?' Yes, like that; these exact words. I said: 'Look, I am here to learn.' So ... well ... (laughs). [...] That hurt me very much"*.

Some supervisees noted the supervisor's irresponsible behaviour: *"It bothered me that once he fell asleep, he smoked, and he was late, he didn't stick to our contract. He didn't inform me in time that he would be late. I was waiting there like ... If he was testing my sense of importance, OK; but this was 15 minutes. He can't just leave me waiting for 15 minutes, can he"?*

" ... Three times she invited me for lunch and then three times she cancelled it. Nonsense".

Supervisee's characteristics, contributing to alliance ruptures

In addition to the supervisors' characteristics, some supervisees' characteristics can also lead to hindering events in the supervision and contribute to alliance ruptures. One of the most evident is the supervisee's feelings of shame and dysfunctional self-critic (Graff, 2008; M. Žvelc, 2017). Both are triggered in a new learning environment and where there is a power difference. Supervision is this kind of situation, so some degree of shame and the presence of the inner critic are inevitable and to be expected in supervisees (Alonso & Rutan, 1988; Graff, 2008; Hahn, 2001; Talbot, 1995). But some supervisees are more prone to harsh shame and self-criticism or have less capacity to cope with them than others. This is related to their attachment style, mindful awareness, self-compassion, and self-regulation abilities. The appearance of shame and self-criticism also depend on the relationship built with the supervisor, so it is a relational phenomenon.

Dysfunctional shame and high internal criticism of the supervisee can immobilise them and compromise their performance during supervision.

They can become passive. If the supervisor does not recognise the supervisee's passivity as a sign of anxiety and shame, they may attribute it to the supervisee's low motivation or resistance, which may lead to a relational impasse.

A supervisee who is prone to self-criticism may project that the supervisor thinks critically of them (Watkins et al., 2022), which may lead to withdrawal or a confrontational supervisory rupture. One supervisee described this inner process of high self-criticism during the supervision session in the following way: *"I feel attacked quickly, and then I say to myself: 'What are you doing? You are completely incompetent; what did you want to say with that? You don't know anything. Awful, explain, correct, you suck ... ' It happened very, very, very, very quickly ... It was so disturbing that I often blocked, froze, stopped; I couldn't say a word"* (M. Žvelc, 2017).

Group characteristics contributing to alliance ruptures

Dysfunctional dynamics in the supervision group, like the hierarchy of power between supervisees, conflict in the group, or an unstable frame, are all connected to supervisory alliance ruptures. With an unstable frame, we refer to group members joining or leaving the group without predictability, changing the time and place of the group meetings, etc. A group may trigger the inner critic and shame processes even more strongly than the dyadic relationship, which can lead to impasses in the supervisory alliance. One supervisee shared her hindering experience in the group with the following words: *"Sometimes I have an idea about what my colleague could do in therapy, and I don't say it out loud because I don't know if my idea would be meaningful for others."* (M. Žvelc & Žvelc, 2021, p. 244).

Based on our research (M. Žvelc, 2017), we have described the main characteristics of the supervisor, supervisee, and the group that can lead to alliance ruptures. Other researchers have detected additional problematic events related to sexuality, sexual attraction, and gender role conflicts within the supervisory relationship (Ladany et al., 2005; Nelson & Friedlander, 2001).

The consequences of problematic relational events in supervision

Supervisees who report hindering events in their supervision sessions are less satisfied with the supervision (Ramos-Sánchez et al., 2002; M. Žvelc, 2017). After a supervision session with hindering events, the supervisees feel incompetent, hurt, angry, ashamed, in shock, frozen, or useless (M. Žvelc, 2017). The following are some examples of supervisees' statements from our research.

"I felt some kind of weight. It was squeezing me; I was left feeling much more burdened and very little of self-esteem; and with this, I went home".

"I felt as if he embarrassed me. I was hurt. It was totally unproductive, and you get nothing from this kind of supervision, absolutely nothing".

"I was shocked; I was feeling completely lousy, I mean, as a therapist".

Because of these problematic events, some of the supervisees left supervision or changed their supervisor. Some supervisees stayed in the same supervisory relationship but showed signs of avoidance: They were less active during supervision sessions, more tense, and less spontaneous. They presented their cases selectively, more likely concealing certain information, and avoiding some topics.

One of the supervisees, for example, concealed in the supervision that: *"The client does not come to my office; we go for long walks instead and have our session during the walk"*. Another supervisee did not disclose in the supervision *"feelings of attraction that I occasionally feel towards the client"* (M. Žvelc & Žvelc, 2021, p. 244).

Some supervisees were selectively using the information and directions from the supervisor. Because of disagreement about the methods and goals of psychotherapy, some were losing their professional identity. In the following statement, the supervisee shares her experience after a supervision session, in which she showed the tape of the psychotherapy session to the supervisor, who disagreed with how she led the psychotherapy. *"I had a very strong feeling of being incompetent … And I was kind of lost, actually. What now? […] This is … This is part of me, that's me, what to do now if I am not allowed to do this"*.

Inadequate or harmful supervision?

Research shows that there is a hindering event in one in every ten supervision sessions (M. Žvelc, 2017). Almost every supervisee, at some point in their career, experiences some conflictual or unproductive event during supervision (Ellis et al., 2014; Gray et al., 2001; Jacobsen & Tanggaard, 2009; Nelson & Friedlander, 2001; M. Žvelc, 2017). This means that problematic events are present during supervision and are probably inevitable.

Ellis et al. (2014) distinguish between inadequate and harmful supervision. Inadequate supervision fails to meet the criteria for minimal adequate supervision: Enhancing the professional functioning of the supervisee, monitoring the quality of their work, and serving as a gatekeeper (Ellis et al., 2014). In such supervision, the supervisor does not attune to the supervisee's professional needs (Ellis, 2001). Inadequate supervision is non-productive but is not harmful. Harmful supervision causes psychological, emotional, or physical harm or trauma to the supervisee and violates ethical standards (Ellis, 2001; Ellis et al., 2014). It may include sexual harassment or sexual intercourse with the supervisee, the supervisor's abuse of power, humiliation, vengeance, violating emotional boundaries, breaking confidentiality, and sexual, homophobic, or racist behaviour towards the supervisee (Ellis, 2001). Ellis et al. (2014) found a striking proportion of supervisees who, from their perspective, are currently receiving inadequate (93%) and harmful (35%)

supervision. In our research (M. Žvelc, 2017), we also found evidence of harmful supervision, mostly related to supervisors' humiliating behaviour and crossing boundaries.

It is important to discuss the problem of harmful supervision, how to prevent it, and how to react to it when it happens. There are different ways to approach this problem, such as educating supervisees about the supervision process and their rights, preparing them to deal with harmful events, improving the supervisors' training, and detecting the supervisors who are more likely to harm the supervisee (Ellis, 2001; Ellis et al., 2014). Our research indicated (M. Žvelc, 2017) that the problematic events were related to ruptures in the supervisory alliance and that the ruptures were not addressed and resolved. We also noticed that both the supervisor and supervisees were unfamiliar with the rupture resolution model (Safran & Muran, 2000; Safran et al., 2008; Watkins et al., 2015). We strongly suggest that it is important to include these themes in all therapeutic and supervisory trainings, regardless of approach. We recommend that the supervisor is mindful of tensions in the supervisory relationship and initiates rupture repair. The supervisor should also make an agreement with the supervisee that they share the responsibility of disclosing, exploring, and resolving ruptures in the supervisory alliance. The supervisor should be sincerely open and ready to talk about the supervisory relationship and be willing to look at their possible mistakes. In this way, bad supervision sessions, which are inevitable, could be prevented from becoming harmful.

Parallel process or supervisory alliance rupture?

Some supervisors, when they detect a difficulty or inconvenience in the supervisory relationship, prematurely conclude that this is a sign of the parallel process and neglect the possibility of a supervisory alliance rupture (M. Žvelc, 2017). Sometimes the supervisors and supervisees interpret the tension in the supervisory relationship as the parallel to the therapeutic process as a defence to avoid conversations about the relational process in the supervision and avoid their contribution and responsibility (Safran et al., 2008). Sometimes there are parallels between the supervisory and the psychotherapeutic relationship, but sometimes there are not (Safran et al., 2008; M. Žvelc, 2017). When there is an impasse in the supervisory relationship, inquiring into the supervisory relationship should come ahead of any exploration into the therapeutic relationship.

Let's look at a concrete case example of the answers given by a particular supervisor/supervisee pair (M. Žvelc, 2017). The supervisor writes on the questionnaire that something is missing after a particular supervision session and that she cannot connect with the supervisee. She concludes that this dynamic from their supervisory relationship is parallel to the therapy process. Based on her hypothesis that it is a parallel process, her interventions are directed only at inquiring into the therapeutic relationship and what the therapist should do in therapy. On the other side, the supervisee conveys that she does not trust the supervisor, that in many things she disagrees with her, that she is withdrawn because of that, and that this has been going on for some time. This clearly indicated to the researchers a supervisory alliance rupture. If a rupture in the alliance is present, work on rupture resolutions is needed first. This means that analysis of the supervision relationship comes before any analysis of the parallel process. Only after that, inquiry into the psychotherapeutic process and giving directions are effective.

Supervisory alliance rupture repair

In this subchapter, we present how ruptures in the supervisory relationship can be resolved. In the following vignette, we present a supervision case, where we followed the model of rupture resolutions (Safran & Muran, 1996, 2000) and adopted it to the supervision process. This case illustrates stages from rupture resolution in practice: Recognising the signs of an alliance rupture, initiating the reflection process, exploring the rupture experience, and the emergence of the supervisee's underlying needs.

"I felt hurt by your words" – A vignette of supervision rupture repair in group supervision

We describe this vignette from the subjective perspective of the supervisor, where the first author of this book was in the role of the supervisor in a supervision group of three supervisees.

During the last two supervision sessions, I felt unusual pressure in my head. It was similar to a headache, but at the same time, different. I was wondering what was going on. I tried to explain to myself that it was because it was late; it was at the end of a long working day. During the supervision of supervision, I mentioned this unusual sensation. The supervisor of my supervision asked me: "*Where do you sit? How are you sitting as a group*"? Initially, I thought to myself: "*What's that got to do with it?!*". It turned out that the question was vital for understanding the supervision process and supervisory alliance.

At the next group supervision, when we were making session contracts, one of the **supervisees, Lana**, said: "*I don't have anything for today. Nothing specific happened. The others can have more time; I am happy to listen today*".

I (the supervisor) thought this avoidance might be the marker of a supervision alliance rupture. I decided to explore it.

Supervisor to the group: *If your client comes to the session and says today I have nothing for the therapy; nothing significant happened; what would you think about their words; what hypothesis would you have; how come they said this?*

Supervisee Nika:	*I would think maybe he wants to talk about something but doesn't feel safe enough.*
Supervisee Julia:	*Maybe there is something in the relationship with the therapist that bothers him.*
Supervisee Lana:	*I would think that maybe something happened in the last therapy session; something that the client did not like, and now he is withdrawing.*
Supervisor:	*Lana, does something that you and the other group members have said refer to you?*
Supervisee Lana:	*Yes, actually, all.*

Although I expected that there was something that bothered Lana, I was surprised that she felt it all applied to her. I asked: "*Can you say more about this? What is it that is troubling you*"? I initiated the exploration of the supervisee's rupture experience (Safran & Muran, 2000).

Supervisee Lana:	*In the last supervision session, when I presented the client with a drug addiction problem, you asked the group what motivates and keeps his girlfriend to be with him. I felt hurt by those words. I heard that something was wrong with her because she was the partner of a drug addict. I have a partner who is struggling with addiction. I felt like I am bad because of that.*
Supervisor:	*Lana, I am glad you told me that … I am very sorry that I hurt you with my words. I guess I was clumsy with my words and unclear. I was interested in how his script combined with her script. It was not my intention to devalue her … and I am not devaluing you because of your relationship.* I was sincere about this. In the last session, I didn't realise that by talking about the client's girlfriend, I was also speaking to Lana. An apology, if sincere with taking responsibility, can be a powerful reparative intervention (Watkins et al., 2015).
Supervisee Lana:	*I felt so incompetent after the last session. I felt I don't deserve to work with clients because I am unworthy.*

Lana was a beginning supervisee. In this developmental stage, supervisees are very critical of themselves and anxious regarding their performance and professional identity (Stoltenberg & McNeill, 2009).

Silence. The other two supervisees and I were listening to Lana carefully and with compassion. She continued:

Supervisee Lana:	*And next to Julia, I feel even more incompetent (Julia was still new to the group; that day was only her third session).*

> *Sorry Julia, I have nothing against you, but when you talk and express with words so properly, I see you as having so much knowledge; it's like everything you say is so right and perfect ... then I feel even more incompetent.*

The reader may guess, between who I was seating. Lana was on my right, and Julia was on my left. And "in-between" was me, and the pressure caught in my head. I hypothesised that the tension in my head might be the embodied sign of Lana's dysregulated emotions like anxiety and feelings of worthlessness, shame, and incompetence.

Since Lana had a good alliance with me and the other member, Nika, until the last session, she was willing to open up and share her feelings with us when invited.

Supervisee Julia
(replying kindly and gently):

Lana if only you knew ... I am not perfect. When I was a teenager, I was on drugs ... I came out ... I used to doubt if I could be a therapist because of my past, but with the help of my personal therapy, I see that it was an important part of my life ... I have become stronger in my struggles to be clean ... Now I see this can also be my strength. And I see that I can help people.

Lana responded compassionately, and the bond with Julia was strengthened. Then Nika shared her vulnerable past when she doubted herself as a therapist. The atmosphere in the room became very compassionate and touching. I, as a supervisor, was surprised at how much the supervisees revealed and how an intense process of repair and stronger connection happened after that first sign of a rupture.

Supervisor: *Thank you for sharing this ... I am touched. We all have something we regret and are ashamed of, the reason we doubt ourselves as therapists. That does not mean that these things make us bad therapists. With awareness, they might help us to understand our clients better. (Silence ...) I see we all are touched. I think we feel much closer now. Before we end ... I suggest having a group hug.*

We made a circle and gave ourselves a kind, open-hearted, compassionate hug. The group supervision alliance was repaired and moved to greater safety and trust. Since then, I have never had a headache again in this group, and the group continued to work very well.

Process of resolutions of supervision ruptures

Figure 5.1 illustrates the dynamics within supervisory alliance ruptures and the possibility of their resolution. As the figure shows, the alliance rupture is triggered by the supervisor, supervisee, or both. From our clinical practice and research (Grant et al., 2012; Gray et al., 2001; Nelson & Friedlander, 2001; M. Žvelc, 2017), we know that it is essential to resolve supervisory alliance ruptures. If not, the following supervision sessions are prone to be ineffective, and the supervisee can become withdrawn, passive, conceal information, or may simply leave the supervision. They can also express their anger by being confrontational and resisting. One of the significant ways of resolving therapeutic ruptures is what is termed metacommunication, the communication about transactions or implicit communication that is taking place in the relationship here and now (Safran, 2003; Safran & Muran, 2000). It is also recommended for use in supervision (Safran et al., 2008; Watkins et al., 2015; M. Žvelc, 2017). The supervisee or the supervisor can initiate the dialogue about what is happening in the supervisory relationship and how they experience it. Based on clinical and research findings (Casement, 2002; Eubanks et al., 2018; Grant et al., 2012; Safran, 2003; Safran & Muran, 2000; M. Žvelc, 2008; M. Žvelc, 2017), we emphasise that the therapist or

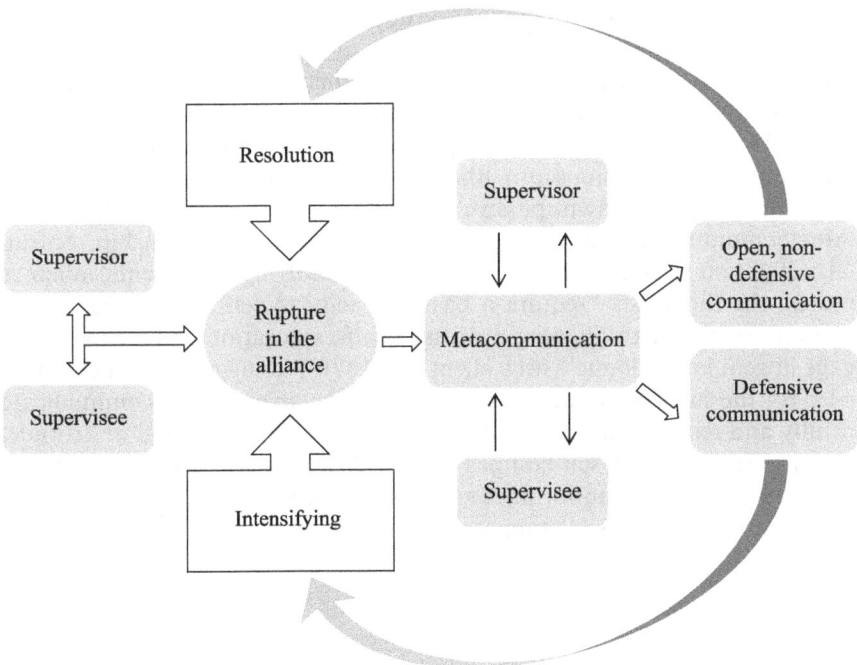

Figure 5.1 Ruptures in supervisory alliance and processes for its resolution.

supervisor should be mindfully attentive to the signs of an alliance rupture, and when they recognise the signs, they initiate metacommunication.

The supervisor in the presented vignette detected the signs of a supervisory alliance withdrawal rupture. The supervisee did not bring a case for presentation and wanted other supervision members to use her time. Based on that sign, the supervisor explored the supervisee's experience by initiating communication about the possible impasse in the supervisory relationship. When the supervisees discussed possible reasons for a client not having a theme for the therapy, the supervisor asked if that was true also for their supervisory relationship.

With initiating communication about their relationship, the supervisor is a model to the supervisees on how they can start the conversation when they are not satisfied with supervision or detect a therapeutic rupture. A part of the supervisory agreement is that possible disagreements and tensions in the supervisory relationship are openly discussed.

If the initiation of metacommunication is followed by open, respectful disclosure by every member about their experience of the supervision and dissatisfied needs, then there is a high chance of resolution of the alliance rupture and its repair. This happened in our vignette; not only was the rupture resolved, but the alliance was re-established at a new level with a greater commitment and bond. The supervisees also experienced a good model of how to deal with therapeutic ruptures.

If one side initiates open communication about the relationship and the other is resistant, attacking, or withdrawing, then resolution and repair are not possible, and the rupture can become even more robust and profound (M. Žvelc, 2017). If there is no metacommunication after the rupture, the following supervisory sessions are likely to be unproductive; the supervisee usually becomes withdrawn, passive or leaves supervision (M. Žvelc, 2017).

Metacommunication depends on all parties to the relationship. Safran et al. (2008) suggest that for the process of resolving therapeutic alliance ruptures, the therapists "require a basic capacity to self-acceptance, a willingness to engage in an ongoing process of self-exploration and a capacity to engage in genuine dialogue with a client" (p. 137). We suggest that the same is needed for the supervisor and the supervisees to be able to meta-communicate fruitfully and resolve supervisory alliance ruptures. For this kind of attitude, mindful awareness and self-compassion are highly important; therefore, in MCIS, we give special importance to both the supervisor's and supervisee's mindful awareness and self-compassion.

Chapter 6

Methods and interventions in integrative supervision

In this chapter, we introduce the integrative model of supervision interventions, which on different taxonomic levels presents methods and interventions of supervision. The model is based on research (M. Žvelc, 2017) and enriched by our clinical experience. The model describes a wide range of supervisor methods and interventions that facilitate supervision change processes, which we present in Chapter 1. The integrative model of supervision interventions is a generic model of supervision that can be used in different supervision approaches.

The integrative model of supervision interventions

The integrative model of supervision interventions is based on a naturalistic study of facilitating and hindering factors in psychotherapy supervision (M. Žvelc, 2015, 2017). The study is based on change process research (Elliott et al., 2001; Elliott, 2010; Greenberg, 1986), using a qualitative design of the helping factors (Elliott, 2010). In the study participated 50 supervisees and their supervisors (N = 12) from different psychotherapy approaches: Integrative psychotherapy, transactional analysis, gestalt therapy, psychoanalytic therapy, systemic therapy, couple and family therapy, and reality therapy. After two supervision sessions, pairs of supervisees and their supervisors were asked to describe the most significant event in their chosen supervision session. Supervisors were also asked about methods and interventions that, in their opinion, led to the significant event. Afterward, the researcher conducted semi-structured interviews with ten supervisees, exploring their supervision experience in depth. Based on qualitative analysis, a model of supervision interventions was developed, which we, in recent years, have elaborated further into the integrative model of supervision interventions (Table 6.1).

This model classifies interventions into seven general categories linked to the various supervision working areas. Within each broad category, there are corresponding subcategories of supervisor interventions.

In this chapter, we explain each category of intervention. By way of illustration, we provide with each category citations from both supervisees

DOI: 10.4324/9781003194118-8

Table 6.1 The integrative model of supervision interventions

Supervision working areas	Subcategories of the supervisor's interventions
1. Interventions directed towards the supervisory relationship **HOW TO RELATE?**	1.1 Interventions focused on establishing the supervisory contract 1.2 The supervisor's respectful and attuned attitude 1.3 The supervisor's openness 1.4 The supervisor's involvement and self-disclosure 1.5 Inquiry about the supervisory relationship 1.6 Working on supervisory rupture repair
2. Interventions focused on the supervisee **HOW TO BE?**	2.1 Inquiry of the supervisee's experience; enhancing mindful awareness 2.2 Validation and normalisation of the supervisee's experience 2.3 Encouraging emotional and physiological regulation 2.4 Promoting the supervisee's self-compassion 2.5 Confirmation of the supervisee and their work
3. Interventions directed towards case conceptualisation **HOW TO UNDERSTAND?**	3.1 Connecting the client's features and the psychotherapy process with the theory 3.2 Interpreting the dynamics of the client, expanding the supervisee's view 3.3 Exploring and reflecting on the meaning of the psychotherapist's counter-transference
4. Interventions focused on psychotherapeutic work **WHAT TO DO?**	4.1 Discussions and suggestions for further work 4.2 Suggestions for further work in connection to the supervisee's countertransference 4.3 Suggestions connected to the psychotherapeutic framework 4.4 Giving clear feedback to the supervisee on their psychotherapeutic work 4.5 Directions connected to ethics and responsibility

5. Working with a supervision group **HOW TO COOPERATE?**	5.1 Working on group atmosphere and group dynamics 5.2 Facilitating supervision group process
6. Activity within the supervisor **WHAT TO DO INTERNALLY?**	6.1 Reflecting on the meaning of the supervisee's (or the client's) behaviour, thinking, emotions, and body reactions 6.2 Mindful awareness and understanding of the supervisor's inner process 6.3 The supervisor's emotional and physiological self-regulation 6.4 Attuning to the supervisee and the client
7. Interventions directed to the **psychotherapeutic and** **supervisory system** **WHERE IS THE PARALLEL?**	7.1 The supervisor's observation and reflection on the supervision process and making possible connections with the therapeutic system

and supervisors from our research (M. Žvelc, 2017), showing the practical use of the interventions.

Interventions directed towards the supervisory relationship: How to relate?

Interventions directed towards the supervisory relationship promote the process of maintaining and repairing the supervisory alliance, which is one of the main mechanisms for change attributed to the interpersonal dimension. The quality of the supervisory alliance is encouraged by the establishment of the supervisory contract, the respectful and attuned attitude of the supervisor, and the supervisor's openness to different views. Supervisees appreciate if their supervisor trusts them and takes them seriously. Inquiry about the supervisory relationship and working on rupture repair are also helpful supervisory methods.

Interventions focused on establishing the supervisory contract

Interventions focused on establishing supervisory contracts include negotiating tasks and goals of supervision. The supervisor noted: "*It was significant that we made a clear supervision session contract because the supervisee was jumping from one theme to another*".

Contracting in supervision is discussed in more detail in Chapter 5.

The supervisor's respectful and attuned attitude

Supervisees state that it is helpful for their development and growth if their supervisor is empathic, attuned, respectful, humble, and present.

> "*For me, it was important that the supervisor was interested in my inner experience, and he encouraged me where I felt weaker and vulnerable*".
> "*I liked that after I told the supervisor my story, he did not come out at once with a theoretical explanation, but he first tried to feel me, where I am*".
> And one of the supervisors stated: "*My supervisee was touched when I noticed her vulnerable part*".

The supervisor's openness

Supervisees value their supervisor's openness toward their different opinions, theoretical backgrounds, and use of methods. This does not mean that the supervisor necessarily agrees but is open to discussion.

> "*It is significant that I can say no to my supervisor's view, that I can discuss this with him; in short, that I can sometimes see something differently, and the supervisor allows this*".

The supervisor's involvement and self-disclosure

Supervisees report that it is valuable and helpful if the supervisor is interested in their work, confirming, supportive, shows emotions, and self-discloses. Supervisors self-disclose some experiences from supervision (for instance, how they are experiencing the supervisee or their client) or some experience from their professional or personal life.

"The supervisor admitted that she is also unfamiliar with the particular topic. Then I realised it is normal to feel fear because that area is new and unknown to me. She helped me to overcome my perfectionist expectations towards myself that I have to master every problem, every client and situation at the first moment".

Inquiry about the supervisory relationship

One powerful supervision method is to inquire about the supervisory relationship. The supervisor may ask the supervisee how they are experiencing their relationship and relationship with other supervision members. For the supervisee, it was significant: *"when the supervisor asked me how it was for me when she told me her feedback on my interventions"*. The supervisor can also self-disclose how they are experiencing the supervisory relationship and may enhance communication about the supervisory relationship with the intervention of *meta-communication* (Safran & Muran, 2000) that involves communication about the present interaction between supervisor and supervisee. This intervention is also significant when the supervisor wants to initiate supervision rupture repair.

Working on supervisory rupture repair

A very significant category of supervision methods involves working with rupture repair, which is treated in more detail in Chapter 5. Let's see one supervisor's statement: *"With this supervisee, often in the past, there were ruptures in our working relationship. Now the relationship has improved, and she is feeling safer. I contributed to that by opening conversations about impasses in our relationship and searching for my part in them"*.

Interventions focused on the supervisee: How to be?

Interventions focused on the supervisee influence the supervisee's way of being in supervision and, consequently, the supervisee's state of mind in the following therapy sessions. They enhance processes of mindfulness and compassion in supervision and promote change processes mostly on affective and physiological dimensions (awareness and acceptance of emotions, emotional regulation, interoception, and physiological regulation).

Inquiry of supervisee's experience; enhancing mindful awareness

One significant intervention is the supervisor's inquiry or acknowledgement of the supervisee's experience in the psychotherapy or supervision session, thereby, enhancing the supervisee's awareness of their own experience. In the following example, the supervisee emphasises the significance of the supervisor's acknowledgement of his behaviour and feelings: *"The supervisor told me that she noticed that at the beginning of the session, I looked absent and restless"*.

Supervisors also describe the importance of enhancing awareness of the supervisee's experience: *"I asked the supervisee to notice her feelings when she talks about the client. More attempts were needed, but she stopped talking about him and spoke up about her fear. After that, a new space opened; it was good"*.

Later in this book, we expand on this theme, especially in Chapter 7, Mindfulness-oriented interventions in integrative supervision.

Validation and normalisation of the supervisee's experience

Supervisees are often anxious or self-critical regarding their feelings toward their clients and the therapy work. Because of shame and expectation of criticism, they often conceal their feelings from the supervisor, especially feelings of dislike, anger, powerlessness, emptiness, despair, or attraction toward the client (M. Žvelc, 2017; M. Žvelc & Žvelc, 2021). If supervisees cannot tolerate their feelings, that leaves them dysregulated and can paradoxically lead to *acting out* instead of reflecting on them in supervision. Supervisees are able to disclose their feelings connected to their client and therapy work if they perceive the supervisor as open and supportive and feel safe in the supervisory relationship (Ladany et al., 1996; Mehr et al., 2010; M. Žvelc & Žvelc, 2021). The supervisor's validation and normalisation of the supervisee's feelings impact the supervisee's acceptance of feelings, their regulation, and possible further exploration of their meaning. This kind of intervention also supports self-acceptance towards the supervisee as a person and can lead to self-compassion. It also increases the possibility that the supervisee will share their feelings in future supervision sessions.

Let us look at one example of validation and normalisation:

"During the therapy session, I became very sad while listening to the client's story and told him that. While reflecting on the transcript in supervision, the supervisor supported my intervention, that I can 'allow' myself these kinds of feelings".

Encouraging emotional and physiological regulation

The emotional and physiological regulation process is very significant in our approach to supervision, and we elaborate on it in detail in Chapters 4 and 9.

Emotional and physiological regulation can be promoted with some of the interventions we have already mentioned, like raising mindful awareness and validation and normalising the experience.

The following example shows how the supervisor's normalisation regulated the supervisee's tension and anxiety caused by her inner critique.

"The supervisor unburdened me from my inner critique that I was doing something wrong. He explained that what I am experiencing is very human and not so rare among therapists. With that, he unburdened me a lot".

One supervisor noted: »*I encouraged the supervisee to allow himself to be with his feeling of uncertainty".*

The supervisor in the following example regulated the supervisee by mindful awareness and acceptance of their feelings: *"When I talked to the supervisee about the message and the meaning of that death of the client's child, I saw, and he also told me, that this is for him too much ... And I could accept this, I respected his feelings and mine ... we allowed ourselves sadness and 'mourning', and the supervision left me in deep peace".* The supervisee from this example told us in the interview that it was hard for him to grieve and live with separations and that until that supervision session, he avoided the theme of the child's death in that couple therapy. The supervision session helped him get in contact with his sadness (which he avoided) and accept it. In the next therapy session, he could open the theme of death, stay present, and be with the parents talking for the whole hour about the child's death and funeral.

Promoting the supervisee's self-compassion

Supervisees are often critical of themselves and their work, or they suffer in other ways connected to their work. This is why encouragement and developing an accepting, kind, and caring relationship towards themselves is needed. The supervisor encouraged the supervisee: *"Imagine yourself back in that last therapy session, when the client was angry at you, and look at yourself with loving eyes. What happens?"*

As promoting self-compassion is one of the main MCIS interventions, we emphasise and explain the processes of promoting self-compassion in Chapters 10 and 11.

Confirmation of the supervisee and their work

It is crucial for supervisees that the supervisor supports them, praises and encourages them, and confirms that they are working well. The statement below from one of the supervisees is typical of many: *"I've got the confirmation that I am doing and thinking in the right way".* These interventions re-establish the supervisee's self-confidence and perception of self-efficiency and regulate the supervisee's emotions and physiology. These interventions may also enhance the supervisory bond.

Supervisees often struggle with self-criticism and anxiety regarding their self-efficacy, especially beginning supervisees (Stoltenberg & McNeill, 2009; Watkins et al., 2022). Their inferences about what the supervisor thinks about their efficiency may be incorrect (Watkins et al., 2022). That is why the supervisor's realistic praise and confirmation are needed.

Supervisors are aware of the significance of these confirmations, too:

"I encouraged the supervisee that she could trust herself and her interventions. She was satisfied and reassured about how to work in the following sessions".

"The supervisee told me about the strategies she used with the client and almost excused herself because that was probably not enough of 'gestalt therapy'. But I praised her and told her that, in my opinion, she was doing right".

Interventions directed towards case conceptualisation: How to understand?

With interventions directed towards the conceptualisation of the case, the supervisor helps the supervisee to conceptualise the case, make a psychotherapeutic diagnosis, and understand the client. These interventions are directed to the cognitive dimension of the supervisee and target two change processes: 1) Understanding a client and the therapeutic process, and 2) Self-reflection and mentalisation.

Connecting the client's features and the psychotherapy process with the theory

Within this category of interventions, the supervisor inquires about the client's experience and connects the client's features, personality, and therapeutic process with the theory. They may also encourage the supervisee to reflect and make theoretical connections themselves. The category also includes discussing diagnosis.

One of the transactional analysis supervisees from the research stated that what was significant for her was: *"the supervisor's illustration of the client's drivers and injunctions and explanation about what holds the client's head above the water so that he does not sink".*

The supervisor can also remind the supervisee regarding a particular theory, or they can explain a piece of theory in supervision: *"The supervisee told me that she liked the theoretical part in the supervision session. She appreciated the illustrated schema, which explains delusions and hallucinations, and why contact with such patients is harder to make".*

Interpreting the dynamics of the client, expanding the supervisee's view

The supervisor's helpful interventions are also interpretations of the client's dynamics and reframing and expanding the supervisee's view. For one supervisee, what was most important in the session was *"when the supervisor explained the emotional dynamics within the couple, that the female client's powerlessness, fear and loneliness is showing in the form of strong anxiety and verbal violence, and the male client is withdrawing".*

Another supervisee liked it when the supervisor helped him *"direct the focus of the treatment from the 'identified client", the child, towards the whole family (also extended) and other significant people for this child. In this way, the view of the 'individual problem' lessened. With redirection on the system, many possibilities opened, and new sources of help, as well".*

In the following example, we see the supervisor's view of the significance of her explanations:

"With the supervisee, we discussed how sometimes some memories within the parents appear at the time when the children are the same age as they were when the trauma happened to them. The client's son was now the same age as the client when the traumatic event occurred. This insight calmed down the supervisee; because before, she was asking herself why the client's fear appeared right now".

Exploring and reflecting on the meaning of the psychotherapist's countertransference

A significant supervisor's intervention concerns exploring and understanding the supervisee's countertransference. The supervisor invites the supervisee to reflect on the meaning of their countertransference response in connection to the psychotherapy process and the client's features, personality, and dynamics.

"When I was describing the therapy case, the supervisor wondered if my anxiety and care towards the client is the consequence of my worry that I, too, would 'betray him and let him down', as significant others in his life had done".

Interventions focused on psychotherapeutic work: What to do?

In this category, the supervisor's interventions help the supervisee evaluate their psychotherapeutic work with the client and determine how to proceed further. These interventions help with treatment planning and direct the supervisee to which methods and interventions to use in the particular therapy. These interventions enhance the processes of change related to the cognitive dimension (understanding and reflection on what to do in psychotherapy) and behavioural dimension (practising the skills).

Discussions and suggestions for further work

The supervisors will here discuss with their supervisees how to proceed with the work and give concrete suggestions. Supervisees often explicitly state how important it is for them when the supervisor directs them, how they should lead the therapy or give them concrete guidance on what to do: "*I asked the supervisor, shall I wait, that the couple start the topic (death of their child) or shall I open this theme; and the supervisor said, yes, start with that theme. And I did*".

The supervisors also identified directions for further work as significant interventions:

> "*Together with the supervisee, we realised that she intervenes too quickly at the therapy sessions; and then we made a deal that she will practise more active listening before making a session contract with the client*".

> "*The significant event in the session was the discussion with the supervisee, how she can let the client know when his behaviour becomes inappropriate during couple therapy (e.g. when he humiliates his wife)*".

Suggestions for further work in connection to the supervisee's countertransference

Helpful interventions are when the supervisor gives suggestions to supervisees on how to deal with their countertransference in the ensuing therapy sessions. The supervisor proposes how the supervisee can use or regulate their experiences in the next psychotherapy sessions.

Let's see some examples from the supervisee's perspective:

> "*For me, his suggestion was significant to stay with my discomfort and observe it while being with the client. (When I am with her, I have difficulties feeling it)*".

> "*With the help of my supervisor, I recognised that I want things to unfold quickly, and I realised that I have to adapt my rhythm to the client's rhythm*".

Suggestions connected to the psychotherapeutic framework

Significant interventions in this category are also directed to the therapy structure or so-called therapeutic frame (Langs, 1994). They include resolving questions or problems over setting boundaries with clients (such as phone calls outside the sessions, difficulties with ending the therapy sessions, changing the time of sessions, irregular attendance, etc.). These interventions often lead the supervisee to self-protect and self-care.

One supervisor stated: *"We touch on the area of the supervisee's self-care; to set the boundaries for her client regarding her irregularity of coming to therapy"*.

The supervisee described the significant moment relating to the psychotherapeutic framework with the following words: *When deciding to postpone the time of the therapy session at the wish of the client, "the supervisor said it is important to understand why specific clients wish to change the therapeutic frame"*.

Interventions often facilitate more than one supervision process. For instance, the above intervention also encourages the supervisee's understanding.

Giving clear feedback to the supervisee on their psychotherapeutic work

This category of intervention includes providing feedback to the supervisee about their work. Concrete feedback, positive and balanced (what was good and what the supervisee needs to change or improve), is required and helpful.

"Very precious for me was the feedback that my self-disclosure was appropriate and supportive, in the right amount, and that I could continue with such interventions in this case".

"The supervisor informed me about my laughter while expressing anger in supervision towards the client".

Directions connected to ethics and responsibility

This significant subcategory includes interventions connected to the question of ethics and supervisees' responsibilities. Discussing the relevant ethical procedures is often needed, and sometimes clear directions are needed from the supervisor. Supervisors may direct the supervisee to personal psychotherapy, suggest the supervisee refers the client to another professional, recommend additional training, give suggestions for resolving dual roles, and other interventions.

Example: *"I alerted the supervisee regarding the client's state and that it would be good that she refers the client to a psychiatrist"*.

Working with a supervisory group: How to cooperate?

In group supervision, the group atmosphere and the activities of the group members are significant factors contributing to the quality of the supervision process (M. Žvelc, 2015). The supervisor's interventions, oriented to the group, are inevitable in the group supervision process. Helpful interventions in this domain are connected to the work on group atmosphere and group dynamics and facilitation of group processes.

Working on group atmosphere and group dynamics

Within this subcategory of interventions, the supervisor introduces the group members, provides a clear group contract and clear information, shares the observation of the group's dynamics, and initiates metacommunication about group relations.

One supervisee wrote: "*We spoke about the group, shared what was bothering us, what we were noticing within the group. I think this was significant for all members of the supervision group*".

Facilitating supervision group process

The supervisor's task is to include all the group members in the supervision work, facilitating comments and feedback from group members, encouraging them to share their experiences, and facilitating group discussion. With discussion, we mean reciprocal and circular deliverance of opinions. The following statements are from the supervisors:

"*The intervention, which led to the helpful event in the session, was asking the group for feedback to the supervisee, who was presenting the case*".

"*I asked members what are they experiencing while they were listening to the case*".

Activity within the supervisor: What to do internally?

This category of activity within the supervisor (M. Žvelc, 2017) is an interesting category of implicit supervisor's tasks, that is seldom mentioned, although Hawkins and Shohet (2012) do describe this theme in their seven-eyed model. This category refers to the supervisor's purposeful mental and mindful activity during the supervision process, which is happening internally inside them. Specifically, it is related to the processes of mentalisation, mindful awareness, emotional and physiological regulation and attunement of the supervisor. This activity is not visible; the supervisee is oblivious to it, except if the supervisor reveals their internal process. Below, we present the main categories of the supervisor's inner activity.

Reflecting on the meaning of the supervisee's (or the client's) behaviour, thinking, emotions, and body reactions

This refers to the supervisor's internal reflection about the meaning of the supervisee's (or the client's) behaviour, thinking, emotions, and body reactions and understanding of their process. These activities are linked to the supervisor's capacity for mentalisation (Fonagy et al., 2004). One supervisor shared in our research his inner activity, which he found significant: "*I was guessing; what kind of supervisee's emotional process or belief could be behind this supervision question*".

Mindful awareness and understanding of the supervisor's inner process

The supervisor is also attentive to their own internal experience: By mindful awareness and reflection on their experience.

"*In the session, it was significant that I followed my inner feelings and was in contact with my emotional processes*".

The supervisor's emotional and physiological self-regulation

Besides mindful awareness and mentalisation of their own experience, the supervisor's important task is their emotional and physiological regulation.

One supervisor noted: "*What was helpful? When I listened to my inner experience and tried to calm down my fear, then I felt more alive*".

Attuning to the supervisee and the client

Another significant inner activity of the supervisor is empathic attunement to the supervisee's experience.

"*I stepped into the shoes of the relatively inexperienced therapist and thought that the supervisee needs affirmations regarding her work*".

"*By listening to the tape, I could understand how it is for my supervisee with this client*".

In addition to attuning to the supervisee, empathic attunement to the client is also a significant activity within the supervisor.

"*First, I tried to immerse myself in the couple's world deeply; I very much sensed the husband*".

"I was empathically attuning to the client's way of thinking and her perception of relationships".

Interventions oriented to the psychotherapeutic and supervisory system: Where is the parallel?

This category encompasses both psychotherapeutic and supervisory systems simultaneously. It includes the supervisor's observation and reflection on the supervision process and making possible connections with the therapeutic system. This category is linked with the concept of the parallel process (Tracey et al., 2012; Watkins, 2012). Within this intervention, the supervisor is considering three supervision subjects: The client, the therapist/supervisee, and themselves. That is why this process can also be called 'triadic'. Processes, which are happening in the course of supervision, can also reflect the processes present in therapy, and vice versa, with the processes in the course of supervision being reflected in the subsequent therapy sessions (Tracey et al., 2012). In the parallel process, the supervisee is an intermediary who carries the reciprocal processes between therapy and supervision. Reflection and understanding of the supervision processes can illuminate the processes in psychotherapy which were unnoticed and not reflected. The supervisor's task is: 1) To mindfully observe their inner process (thoughts, emotions, body sensations, and behaviour) and processes in the supervisee and supervisory relationship, 2) To reflect and to look for meanings about possible connections with the therapy, and 3) Based on this reflection, intervene in supervision (for instance sharing and discussing their hypothesis about the parallel process with the supervisees).

In the following excerpt, the supervisor assumes that her supervision experience is connected to the therapy system. In this intervention, she considers all three supervision subjects: The client, the supervise, and herself. *"While presenting the case, I experienced my supervisee in a quite different way than usual. He became quieter and withdrawn; I did not recognise him. I told him this. When I was listening to the client's life, I was becoming angry and agitated. Then I asked the supervisee how this client reminds him of himself. The supervisee deepened the contact with himself and became vulnerable. Then I calmed down, and we could discuss the therapy process with genuine vulnerability and come into closer contact between ourselves".*

The parallel was that the supervisee was withdrawing from contact with the client and his inner contact, and while presenting the case, also withdrawing from contact with the supervisor. The supervisor was becoming angry like the therapist was in the psychotherapy session. In the supervision session, the supervisor did something different from the supervisee; she did not avoid her internal process (anger) or step back from contact with the supervisee. She was modelling presence, regulation, and how to stay in contact. This new experience the supervisee internalises and brings to the following therapy session.

In Chapter 3, we presented the mindfulness- and compassion-oriented transformative supervision model, where we propose that a significant component of the parallel process is the supervisee's implicit relational schema of being with the client. In MCIS, in addition to understanding and reflecting on the parallel process, we promote the transformation of relational schemas of being with the client with the help of mindful awareness and self-compassion. Transformed relational schemas influence the supervisee's experience of the client in subsequent psychotherapy sessions.

Processes appearing in the course of supervision are not necessarily parallel to the therapy process. Sometimes supervisors conclude prematurely that a parallel process is occurring and neglect other possibilities, such as rupture in the supervisory alliance (M. Žvelc, 2017) (see Chapter 5).

The integrative model of the supervisor's interventions in the context of supervision research

The integrative model of the supervisor's interventions is based on change process research of significant events in supervision (M. Žvelc, 2015, 2017). The categories of interventions from the model are comparable and supported by other studies. The meaning of the supervisory relationship with a respectful, empathic, supportive, and open supervisor who also sometimes self-discloses was found in various studies (such as Allen et al., 1986; Carter et al., 2009; Henderson et al., 1999; Hutt et al., 1983; Jacobsen & Tanggaard, 2009; Knox et al., 2008; Martin et al., 1987; Rabinowitz et al., 1986; Strozier et al., 2000; Worthen & McNeill, 1996). As in our research, Allen et al. (1986), Carter et al. (2009), Jacobsen and Tanggaard (2009), and Worthington and Roehlke (1979) showed the significance of the conceptualisation of the cases and connection of cases with theory. We also found the importance of the supervisor's directions for the ensuing psychotherapeutic work, which is congruent with the findings of other authors (Carter et al., 2009; Rabinowitz et al., 1986; Worthington & Roehlke, 1979). Our research is congruent with the authors, who found the significance of clear supervisor feedback, learning practical skills (Allen et al., 1986) and exploration and understanding of the supervisee's experiences connected to the psychotherapy with the client (Carter et al., 2009; Jacobsen & Tanggaard, 2009; Rabinowitz et al., 1986; Rožič, 2018). Regarding group supervision, other researchers also found the significance of establishing safety in a group and the meaning of other members' activities (Carter et al., 2009; Jacobsen & Tanggaard, 2009; Ögren et al., 2002).

The empirically based categories from our study significantly overlap with Hawkins and Shohet (2012) seven-eyed model. The seven-eyed model is recognised and widely used in supervision training and clinical practice. We find particularly helpful Hawkins' and Shohet's (2012) division of two matrixes in supervision: The client-therapist matrix and the supervisee-supervisor matrix. The supervisor may focus on either of them in supervision.

In our model, the client-therapist matrix is related to interventions oriented towards the conceptualisation of the case and interventions oriented towards psychotherapy work. Interventions in our model that mainly focus on the supervisee-supervisor matrix are: Interventions oriented toward the supervisory relationship, interventions oriented towards the supervisee, working with the supervisory group, and activity within the supervisor. The category of interventions that are directed to the psychotherapeutic and supervisory systems simultaneously is related to both matrixes.

The use of the model in supervision practice and training

The integrative model of the supervisor's interventions is trans-theoretical and relevant for supervision from different approaches. It presents guidelines for supervisors for their actions. We suggest that flexible use of these interventions is needed for effective supervision. As supervisors, we attune to what is needed at a particular moment in supervision. Sometimes understanding the client may be central; at other times, interventions focused on the supervisory alliance. The focus of interventions depends on the supervisory contract and what is most salient in the supervisory process.

Based on the model, supervisors can also reflect on which interventions they use more frequently and which category of intervention they may seldom use. If they realise they are not skilled in using certain interventions, they might further educate themselves in that direction. From our experience in teaching supervision, some, even established supervisors, realise that they use interventions only from certain categories (for instance, from cognitive and behavioural dimensions) and want to learn more about the use of other interventions as well (for example, relational or emotional). Integrative supervision emphasises the comprehensive and holistic use of all interventions.

The use of interventions also depends on the supervisee's developmental level. Supervisees at the start of their professional development experience higher anxiety and self-doubt and are searching for their professional identity. Compared to more advanced supervisees, they need more support, confirmation, and directions on how to lead therapy (Erskine, 1982; Stoltenberg & McNeill, 2009; M. Žvelc, 2017).

The model can also be helpful in supervision training. We often divide trainees into smaller groups. Each small group is then given the task of writing a few specific statements, which the supervisor can concretely say or do in relation to a particular category of interventions. Next to each category of interventions, the groups then write two or three concrete sentences for the supervisor. For instance, next to the subcategory "validates and normalises the supervisee's experience" (listed in the category Interventions focused on the supervisee), the group writes concrete sentences the supervisor may say, such as: "*The anger you are feeling in the therapy with this client has a significant meaning*". The groups then share their written statements. The whole group is enriched by a set of concrete, specific supervisor statements.

Another way of using the model in training is to do a live demonstration of supervision and ask the trainees to check which interventions the supervisor uses.

Conclusion

In mindfulness- and compassion-oriented integrative supervision, we use a broad spectrum of interventions. We want to use them flexibly based on what is needed at a particular moment in the supervision process. Interventions from different areas of supervision are required. In this book, we focus mainly on interventions oriented towards the supervisee, the supervisory relationship, and the activities within the supervisor. In MCIS, we especially emphasise mindfulness- and compassion-oriented interventions and interventions focused on emotional and physiological regulation in supervision. They are central to our supervision approach and are not sufficiently elaborated in the supervision literature.

Part 2

Mindfulness- and compassion-oriented methods in supervision

Chapter 7

Mindfulness-oriented interventions in integrative supervision

The effectiveness of supervision and related clinical practice is significantly enhanced if the supervisee and the supervisor are in a *mindful state of consciousness* (G. Žvelc & Žvelc, 2021) during the supervision session. This chapter presents various methods and interventions that promote mindful awareness during supervision sessions. We present exercises for mindful preparation for supervision and relational methods that promote core mindfulness processes in supervision: Present moment awareness, acceptance, and decentred perspective. We also present examples of mindfulness-oriented interventions directed to different dimensions of the supervisee's experience: Physiological, affective, cognitive, behavioural, relational, and spiritual. The use of mindfulness-oriented interventions is illustrated with the help of two vignettes from our supervision practice.

Mindful preparation for supervision

At the beginning of the session, the supervisor and supervisee(s) may implement a mindful exercise. This prepares them to become more present and in contact with themselves and each other. Such exercises may facilitate openness to their body and emotional processes instead of focusing only on intellectual understanding (Safran et al., 2009). We propose a quick body scan, which involves mindful awareness of body sensations and parts of the body in a gradual sequence from feet to head. We also use 1) The diamond of mindful awareness exercise and 2) The mindful supervision intention exercise.

Exercise: The diamond of mindful awareness

The diamond of mindful awareness (G. Žvelc & Žvelc, 2021) involves mindful awareness of the body, emotions, thoughts, and perceptions of the external environment. The exercise also invites awareness of the observing self. We use the shortened, five-minute version of the exercise:

> *"Becoming aware of your breathing—each in-breath and out-breath. Becoming aware of where you feel the breathing in your body. Maybe you feel it more in*

DOI: 10.4324/9781003194118-10

your nostrils, chest or stomach. (pause) Now bringing attention to the whole of your body. Simply becoming aware of the sensations that might be present. There is no need for changing them or doing anything about them. If you can, allowing them to be as they are. (pause)

Now moving the focus of attention to your emotions. Noticing if there are any emotions present for you right now. If there are, just making space for them and welcoming them all. It is OK as it is. (pause)

Now turning attention to your thoughts. Being aware of each thought coming and going. Becoming aware of the tendency to either cling to or avoid specific thoughts. Just allowing them to be as they are, a passing event in our minds, continually arising and disappearing. (pause)

You are aware of body sensations, emotions and thoughts. Notice that there is someone or something aware of all these .... Become aware of awareness itself. (pause)

Now bringing attention to the external environment. Noticing sounds arising and disappearing. (pause)

Now bringing attention to your body. Becoming aware of your posture as you sit in the chair and the points of contact with the chair. (pause)

As we are coming to the end of this practice, opening your eyes (if they were closed) and looking at the room ... . Trying to see the room with fresh eyes as if seeing it for the first time just now ... .

When this exercise is done in supervision groups, we invite participants to look at each other; if not, the supervisee is invited to look at the supervisor.

Look at your colleagues as if seeing them for the first time in your life. Becoming aware that there is a presence of awareness in each one of you. And when you catch another person's gaze, becoming aware that you are both seeing each other from the place of awareness itself".[1]

Exercise: Mindful supervision intention

The mindful supervision intention exercise can raise mindfulness, compassion, and contact with a spiritual dimension related to getting in touch with inner values. The supervision group spends a few moments at the start of the supervision session to become aware of the intention of the supervision session.

The supervisor may say:

"Becoming aware of the intention of why we are here. We are here, with the noble intention, to do good, to help ... in a way in an amount, that we can ... We can embrace our clients and all of us here, in our imagination, with the awareness of our intention".

Mindfulness during the supervision session

In MCIS, the supervisor continuously and mindfully tracks their own inner states and mindfully observes the supervisee(s). Based on both observations, the supervisor reflects and mentalises, trying to understand the meaning of their own and their supervisees' inner states and, based on that, decides on the further steps in supervision. The supervisor's next task is to lead the supervisee(s) to become mindful of their emotional and bodily experience in supervision, helping to regulate their dysregulated physiology and emotions and reflect on the meaning of their states.

In addition to what the supervisor does externally, what they do internally inside themselves is also vital. One of the essential inner activities of the supervisor is to *be mindfully aware of their inner states:* Their body sensations, emotions, thoughts, and fantasies here and now in the supervision. This awareness of the supervisor's own internal state may inform the supervisor about implicit, but not yet verbalised processes in the supervision and a possible parallel process. The supervisor also mindfully listens to the content and, at the same time, *mindfully observes the supervisee's nonverbal signs.* The changes in the supervisee's body reflect the changes in their physiology. The physiology of the supervisee often holds important information about the supervision and therapy process. In the process of mindful observation, the supervisor uses the diamond model of mindful awareness and the triangle of relationship to inner experience (see Chapter 2). These models help the supervisor to assess: 1) Which process of mindful awareness they need to enhance: Present moment awareness, acceptance, or decentred position, and 2) To which dimension of human experience they need to bring mindful awareness. Based on this observation of the supervisee, the supervisor *leads the supervisee to mindful awareness* of their inner states. The supervisor encourages mindful awareness with relational mindfulness-oriented interventions, which help the supervisee to become aware of the present moment, accept their experience, and take a decentred perspective on their experience. With these interventions, the supervisee is invited to relate to their experience from the position of the loving witness.

Promoting mindful awareness in the supervision session

In Chapter 2, we introduce the *keyhole model of relational mindfulness and compassion* that includes three main methods: Inquiry, attunement, and involvement (see Figure 2.3). These three methods encourage the core mindful processes: Awareness of the present moment, acceptance, and decentred perspective.

Promoting present moment awareness in supervision

Promoting present moment awareness is the main process related to mindful awareness and invites the supervisee to become aware of their current experience in the supervision process. We promote the supervisee's present moment awareness by *phenomenological inquiry* and *acknowledgement* of the supervisee's experience (G. Žvelc & Žvelc, 2021). In MCIS, we regularly bring the attention of the supervisee to the present moment with inquiries related to the fundamental dimensions of human experience (body sensation, emotions, cognitions, behaviour, relationships, and spiritual dimension). The supervisor may inquire and ask the supervisee about their here-and-now experience: *"What are you experiencing in your body now?", "What are you feeling now?", "Are there any thoughts or images which are going through your mind?", "What are you experiencing in the relationship with me?"*

In addition to inquiry, present moment awareness is also promoted by the supervisor's *acknowledgement* of the supervisee's experience. By acknowledging a particular aspect of the supervisee's experience, the supervisee is invited to become aware of their experience in the present moment. Acknowledgement may involve empathic reflection: *"It seems you are feeling very scared of your client.", "I sense a lot of pain when you discuss the client who lost her mother"*. It may also involve bringing attention to overt but non-verbal body behaviour: *"When discussing your client's break up in their partnership, I notice that you talk with a louder voice than usual"*.

Facilitating acceptance of the supervisee's experience

In the keyhole model of relational mindfulness and compassion, the main methods for facilitating acceptance are 1) *validation* and 2) *invitation to the supervisee to willingly attend to their experience* (G. Žvelc & Žvelc, 2021). Acceptance of internal experience is an antidote to the supervisee's avoidance of internal experience. It is the primary process used when the supervisor assesses that the supervisee is distanced from their inner experience.

Erskine et al. (2023) describe validation as acknowledging the significance of the person's experience. Validation conveys to the supervisee that their experience is valuable and significant. The supervisor may say: *"This is an important sensation (feeling, thought …). It has a meaning.", "These thoughts about your client are not random; they are telling something important about your relationship.", "I understand your pain; it is tough to sit with the client who is mourning the loss of a relationship"*.

In addition to words, validation is also conveyed through the supervisor's nonverbal communication of acceptance of the supervisee's processes. The supervisor conveys their acceptance through the warm and accepting look of their eyes, voice, facial expression, and gestures.

The invitation to willingly attend to the experience encourages the supervisee to attend to their experience and stay with it instead of running away from it. This helps to develop the supervisee's ability to contain and tolerate difficult internal experiences, which is also an essential ingredient of effective emotional regulation. When the supervisee comes into contact with difficult

experiences, the supervisor may invite the supervisee to focus on that experience and to make space for it: *"Just focus on that sensation in your
stomach."*, *"Let's stay a few moments with this feeling of fear, if you are
willing."*, *"Just allow to come whatever needs to come."*, *"Just attend to your
sensations and observe them"*.

Promoting decentred perspective in supervision

When the supervisee is merged with their experience, we may use different
interventions that invite them to establish a decentred perspective. One of the
most common interventions is the *acknowledgement of experience* and *invitation
to observe their experience mindfully* (G. Žvelc & Žvelc, 2021). The supervisor
may say: *"This is just a sensation (feeling, thought) that you have. Observe it with
curiosity. It may have a significant meaning."*, *"You are feeling lots of fear regarding your client. Just take a few moments and observe how your fear manifests
in your body."*, *"You are having a thought that you are a bad therapist. Just
observe that thought as a cloud on the sky, coming and going."*.

In MCIS, we often use a *language of parts of self* to promote this decentred
perspective. When we label a particular experience of the supervisee as a part,
they may start to relate towards that part from a decentred perspective: *"A
part of you feels like you have to do more in therapy, even in a way that would
go outside of professional boundaries. Take a moment and observe that part of
you. How does it look? Let that part know that you are there and listening to it.
What does this part of you need?"*

Contacting the observing self naturally brings a decentered perspective (see
Chapter 2). The observing self is an aspect of ourselves from which we
observe and experience ourselves and the world. One intervention that helps
the supervisee to decentre from merging with the client is an invitation to
observe an aspect of the psychotherapy session from a third-person perspective. The supervisor may say: *"Just imagine that you are now in the
psychotherapy room with your client when this event happened. Just look at the
client. And now look at yourself. Now, look at both of you at the same time.
What are you experiencing when you are observing yourself with your client?
What do you notice?"*

Sometimes the supervisee may imagine that they are looking at the session
from the perspective of the wise supervisor. *"Imagine that you are a wise
supervisor with many years of experience. Just look at that event in the psychotherapy session through the eyes of the wise supervisor. What do you notice?
What would you say to yourself from this perspective?"*

Awareness of the observing self brings a broader perspective and helps
to decentre. When the supervisee is observing the content of their experience, the supervisor may invite the supervisee to become aware of the
source of awareness itself: *"So you are aware of your anxiety in your chest.
Become aware of the awareness itself. There is something that is observing*

the sensation. What do you experience?" or *"Just ask yourself – who or what is aware?"* Such interventions promotes the ability to contain difficult experiences and observe from a safe perspective. As the observing self is a perspective from which we are watching, it is untouched and not contaminated by experiences. It is a safe place that is always with us; we are just unaware of it most of the time. It is a context in which all our thoughts, emotions, and bodily sensations appear. Because of this, awareness of the observing self helps supervisees to both contain their experience and to self-regulate.

In MCIS, we may use several other interventions to develop a decentred perspective, such as externalisation of inner experience, inquiring about physical properties of experience, and exercises in mindful observation (G. Žvelc & Žvelc, 2021).

Mindfulness-oriented supervisory interventions directed to different dimensions of the supervisee's experience

Mindfulness-oriented supervisory interventions can be directed to different dimensions of human experience in supervision: Physiological, affective, cognitive, behavioural, relational, and spiritual. The diamond model of the observing self (Figure 2.1, Chapter 2) helps the supervisor to determine which dimension of human experience lacks mindful awareness and needs to be attended to. For example, if the supervisee lacks mindful awareness of emotions, the supervisor may invite the supervisee to become aware of their emotions with acceptance.

Mindfulness-oriented interventions directed to the physiological dimension

In MCIS, we stress the primary importance of the embodied awareness of the supervisee and supervisor and the importance of bottom-up processes in supervision. Contact with the body/physiological dimension is seen as the primary process in supervision, from which new cognitive insights emerge. Mindful awareness of the physiological dimension enhances two primary processes related to the physiological dimension: Interoception and physiological regulation (see the integrative model of processes of change, Table 1.1, Chapter 1).

Interventions directed to the physiological dimension raise mindful awareness of body sensations, needs, and movement here and now during the supervision session. The supervisor leads the supervisee to mindful awareness and contact with the body dimension with the use of inquiry or acknowledgement of body sensations, intentions or movement: *"What are you noticing in your body now?", "While talking about your clients, how does your body respond here and now?", "Where in the body do you feel that?", "I hear your voice is shaking while you talk about ...", "I see you stopped breathing ...", "Could you pause for a moment and be aware of your breathing".*

Anchoring the supervisee's mindful awareness in the body is the primary step in supervision. Mindful awareness of the body enables groundedness and presence. Based on it, a supervisee can reflect on the meaning of information coming from their body. Mindful awareness of the body, therefore, enhances interoception, a »process of receiving, accessing, and appraising internal bodily signals" (Farb et al., 2015, p. 1). It also allows the supervisee to come into contact with emotions. Mindful body awareness helps the supervisee recognise their physiological arousal level. This gives them a clue if physiological regulation is needed.

Mindfulness-oriented interventions directed towards the affective dimension

With interventions directed towards the affective dimension, we raise mindful awareness of emotional processes present here and now in the supervision session. These interventions promote processes of change related to the affective dimension: Awareness and acceptance of emotions and emotional regulation (see the integrative model of processes of change, Chapter 1, Table 1.1).

Interventions of inquiry and acknowledgement of emotions enhance mindful awareness of emotional processes within the supervisee. The supervisor encourages the supervisee's observation, acceptance, and decentred perspective towards their emotions. With the validation of emotions (such as *"this is an important feeling"*), they give importance to the emotions here and now and help the supervisee accept them. With validation, they additionally direct supervisees to use mentalisation processes to understand their states. Mindful awareness of emotions also promotes emotional regulation.

Below are examples of emotion-focused mindfulness-oriented supervisory interventions. The following interventions can also raise awareness of body states because emotional states are connected to physiological processes: *"What are you experiencing while talking about your last therapy session?", "Feeling shame (guilt, anger, sadness) while talking about the therapy with your client is important. It holds significant information about the therapeutic relationship.", "While talking about your client, which emotion are you feeling (right now)?"* Combined with the body dimension, we can ask: *"Where do you feel it?"*

If the supervisee is detached from emotions, we explore the meaning of detachment or use interventions to bring them into contact with themselves. Sometimes an exploration of the supervisory alliance is needed; the supervisee might not disclose their emotion because they do not feel safe in the supervisory relationship.

Mindfulness-oriented interventions directed to the cognitive dimension

Mindfulness interventions directed to the cognitive dimension enhance processes of change related to 1) Understanding the client and the therapeutic process and 2) Self-reflection and mentalisation.

Mindfulness interventions in supervision are oriented towards raising the supervisee's mindful awareness of thoughts, judgments, memories, images, fantasies, and ideas.

> *"Do you have any parallel thoughts (images, sounds or fantasies) which are running through your mind now while we are discussing the last therapy session?"*

> *"You are feeling lots of emotions regarding the last session with the client. Just take a short pause and, for a moment, observe your thoughts coming and going through your mind".*

Encouraging mindful awareness with promoting decentred position helps the supervisee to step back from the content of their mind and reflect on it.

After decentred observation of thoughts, the supervisor may encourage meta-cognitive processes: *"How do you understand this?"*, *"What do you think is behind that thought (image, sound, phantasy) that you have? There may be a significant meaning behind it."*, *"How do those thoughts relate to your work with the client?"*.

Such interventions enhance the supervisee's metacognitive processes: Self-reflection and mentalisation. They enable the supervisee to understand what is behind their and their client's mental states. They also help conceptualise the case and think about strategies for further work.

Mindfulness-oriented interventions directed to the behavioural dimension

Mindfulness interventions directed to the behavioural dimension help the supervisee to bring mindful awareness to their behaviour in supervision and to stay present while practising new skills. These interventions are an important component of the deliberate practice (Rousmaniere, 2017) of mindfulness skills in supervision. Supervisees may practise new skills related to learning new interventions and methods. In MCIS, we especially focus on skills related to the internal activity of the supervisee: Mindful awareness and physiological and emotional regulation. While supervisees present the case verbally or through audio or videotapes of psychotherapy sessions, we stop them at significant moments. Supervisees are then invited to raise the mindful awareness of their inner experience and physiologically and emotionally regulate if needed. In this way, they practise new ways of responding to the client.

Practising new skills may also be done through role-playing, where supervision members play either the role of the client or therapist. Mindfulness interventions invite the supervisee to mindful awareness while practising a particular intervention or method. The supervisor may ask the supervisee to pause and observe what they are experiencing while they are practising a specific method or intervention. Alternatively, they may instruct the supervisee to be mindful while performing a specific task: "*While you do this task, pay simultaneous attention to your inner experience*". Such interventions enable the supervisee to learn to maintain mindful awareness during psychotherapy sessions.

In MCIS supervision training, when supervisees deliberately practice skills through role-playing, we sometimes use a bell to indicate the time for mindful awareness of the present moment. When trainees hear the bell, they pause and become mindfully aware of their present experience. In this way, they are experientially learning to maintain mindful awareness of themselves while being in supervision or therapy.

Mindfulness-oriented interventions directed towards the supervisory relationship

Mindfulness interventions directed towards the supervisory relationship encourage the supervisee to become aware of how they are feeling in the relationship with the supervisor or the supervision group and to express their experience. The supervisor inquires about the supervisory relationship and acknowledges the supervisee's experience and behaviour in the supervisory relationship: "*How do you feel in the group?*", "*How do you experience our interaction now?*", "*I notice you are looking away from me*".

The supervisor may also invite the supervisee to observe what is happening at the moment in the supervisory relationship from a decentred perspective:

"*Let us just take a pause and observe what is happening between us right now from a bird's eye perspective. What do we notice?*"

Such mindful interventions are then a starting point for self-reflection and mentalisation about the supervisory relationship. They may help to reveal ruptures in the supervisory relationship (see Chapter 5) or a possible parallel process. In the case of an alliance rupture, the supervisor may use metacommunication, which could be described as *mindfulness in action* (Safran & Muran, 2000).

"*I observe that I feel tense right now when you say that supervision is not helpful and that we are both trying to prove to ourselves that we are competent. What do you experience when I say that?*"

Mindful interventions related to the supervisory relationship are also the starting point for awareness of the parallel process between psychotherapy and supervision. The supervisor may invite the supervisee to reflect:*"Do you see any connection between what we are experiencing in our relationship with your psychotherapy with the client?"*

Mindfulness interventions related to the supervisory relationship enhance the process of maintaining and repairing the supervisory alliance and may reveal a possible parallel process between psychotherapy and supervision.

Mindfulness-oriented interventions directed towards the spiritual dimension

Mindfulness-oriented supervisory interventions directed towards the spiritual dimension refer to the awareness of the spiritual quality of the present moment in supervision. They enhance the processes of 1) Contact with values and meaning and 2) Contact with the observing/transcendent self.

As MCIS is based on mindfulness and compassion, supervisees can sometimes have spontaneous spiritual experiences in the supervision process. Mindfulness and compassion are at the core of different spiritual traditions, and their use is often related to the spiritual path. Inviting supervisees to embrace their experience with mindful awareness and kindness can result in experiences related to higher meaning and contact with the essential transcendent self. The observing/transcendent self is boundless and spacious awareness, a context in which all our thoughts, emotions, and bodily sensations appear (see Chapter 2). Inviting supervisees to become aware of the observing self may result in profound spiritual experiences of interconnection and oneness with other people and nature. Such interventions may be simply invitations to become aware of awareness: *"Just become aware of who is aware? Who is observing your thoughts, emotions and sensations?"* or *"Just take a moment and immerse yourself in the experience of being present – the experience of I am"*. The experience of self-compassion and compassion for others is often related to experiences of interconnection and love that are often felt as profound spiritual experiences.

Mindfulness-oriented interventions may deepen the supervisee's contact with their values related to their psychotherapy work. Values guide our lives and give our life meaning and purpose (Luoma et al., 2007). The following vignette with supervisee Andrew shows how supervision enhanced his awareness of the spiritual dimension related to his broader meaning in life.

Vignette: Coming into touch with meaning and purpose

Andrew comes to the triadic online supervision exhausted, with pain in his lower back. He presents the therapy with a very busy client, who has no time for himself, working overlong hours, and is drained and deprived of his strength and vitality. Andrew says that the rhythm in the therapy is fast, the client is agitated, and Andrew, especially in the last few therapy sessions, had difficulties slowing down and regulating the client. Andrew's pace of talking during the supervision session is accelerated, and he does not seem to be in touch with his body and emotions. While listening to Andrew, the supervisor feels agitated and notices her sympathetic arousal (faster heartbeat, restless limbs). We can see here that a physiological parallel process is being activated in the supervision session; the physiologically dysregulated field from the psychotherapy session was almost at once transferred to the supervision session. The supervisor hypothesises that Andrew has difficulties regulating his and the client's physiology during the psychotherapy. The supervisor concludes she will initiate a *mindful pause* to make a time and space for mindful awareness and physiological regulation. She says: "*Andrew, let's pause for a moment, and let's all three of us notice what we are feeling in our bodies*". She specifically included in the intervention the other supervision member.

Andrew pauses and says: *I feel tiredness in my body, pain in my back, my body is restless.*

Then he looks up, gazing at something. His expression changes, softens; he takes his time to observe something. He is somewhere else; he has entered a different state. The pace slowed down profoundly.

The supervisor feels the significance of this gaze and this change; and says: "*I see you are looking at something*". She imagines that Andrew is looking at some flying birds. She cannot see what he is seeing because the session is online.

Andrew: *There is a bird … Flying. So calm … so steady … she knows the direction, and at the same time, she is so content, free, light … in this vast sky.*

The supervisor takes her time to breathe and imagine the bird, too, and gives space for Andrew to centre himself by observing the bird. A spiritual quality enters the supervision space.

After some time, the **supervisor** asks: "*How would you connect the experience of observing the bird, which flies with ease, dignity, and is free- to the therapy with your client?*"

Using the bird as a resource deepened the spiritual dimension in the supervision session as it brought the supervisee into touch with his inner values – his meaning and purpose.

Andrew slowly answers: *I think we both, my client and I, are lost to some extent. We need to slow down. (pause) It seems that we have lost touch with ourselves. We need to see the wider dimension in our life, what it is really worth.*

His voice, look, and words are all reminiscent of a touch of the spiritual dimension of life. The supervisor and the other supervisee are touched, too, contemplating the meaning his words have for them. Andrew gained a valuable insight that both he and the client are with their preoccupation endlessly hurrying and losing contact within themselves, with others, and with what matters to them. Andrew's state of mind was changed, regulated, and present; with this different state of mind and new insight, he was able to enter the following therapy session differently.

Vignette: Mindful body awareness in supervision

In the following vignette, we present the use of mindfulness-oriented interventions in supervision which lead to present moment awareness, acceptance of the experience, and decentred perspective. The interventions help the supervisor and the supervisee to observe their experience and reflect on them from the position of the *loving witness* (see Chapter 2). The supervisor frequently in the session uses body-oriented mindfulness interventions, which lead the supervisee to embodiment and presence. From this embodied, mindful state, the supervisee is open to further exploration, reflection, and learning.

Therapists Helene and Laura attend ongoing online triadic supervision. Helene presents the psychotherapy case with her client Angela. Helene explains that Angela avoids talking about deeper personal stuff, wanting to amuse with stories from her current life and turning her attention to the therapist asking her about her life. Angela's rhythm of talking is fast, and it seems that Angela is controlling the flow of the therapy session. The therapist, Helene, has difficulties slowing down the rhythm and leading Angela into contact with herself. In the supervision session, Helene describes all this at an accelerated pace. The parallel process has already begun. The client talks fast; similarly, the supervisee talks faster than her usual rhythm without letting herself breathe. In the meantime, the supervisor feels tense in her body and restless in her lower legs. She decides to initiate a *mindful pause*, where supervisees and herself direct mindful awareness to their bodies in this particular moment.

Supervisor: *Helene, may I stop you for a moment? What are you feeling in your body now? Laura, let's both of us also look at what we are experiencing in our bodies.*

The supervisor initiates this mindful pause and interoceptive awareness for the following reasons: 1) She wants Helene to become aware of her body and physiological processes and their possible dysregulation; 2) To help Helene regulate; 3) To lead Helene to explore the meaning of her bodily reactions and gain insight into the possible physiological parallel process, which will help her to understand the psychotherapy process; 4) To model Helene how to slow down the pace, regulate herself and the client, and lead a client into contact with herself. Based on these processes, Helene could enter subsequent therapy with a client with a changed state of mind and lead the therapy differently.

The supervisor also invites the other supervisee, Laura, to mindful awareness because she is part of the supervision intersubjective field. She is reacting to her fellow supervisee's story and physiology. Laura's awareness of body sensations is also an important element that may help them understand the presented therapy case.

Let's see what the supervisees noticed in their bodies.

Supervisee Helene:	*My body is trembling.*
Supervisor:	*I also started to feel trembling soon after you started talking about the client. What do you think? What meaning does it have? You talk about Angela, and your body starts to tremble.*
Supervisee Helene:	*I would say this is the client's state in general in psychotherapy. She has a mask, she is very attractive, but underneath I feel her tense.*
Supervisor:	*Where do you feel trembling?*
Supervisee Helene:	*Mostly here* (showing with her hand her chest), *in the lungs, in the oesophagus, yes.*
Supervisor:	*Laura, and you?*
Supervisee Laura:	*At the beginning, it seemed to me that I didn't feel anything; this is typical of me, that I connect with the strong part, the facade, and now when you start to talk, my back feels freezing cold. And I am gritting my teeth.*
Supervisee Helene:	*Interesting! She has big problems with her teeth.*
Supervisee Laura:	*The client's style of functioning is very close to mine; to be outwardly strong and hide the gentle, vulnerable feminine part, expecting attack or danger.*
Supervisor:	*Splitting is also visible in your body experience, Laura; on one side feeling nothing, and then feeling such intense coldness.*
Supervisee Helene:	*Yes, my client is like that. All or nothing: comes to the therapy and everything is great, or she comes totally crushed.*

Here we can see how all three supervision participants react in their bodies to Helene's presentation of psychotherapy with Angela. As we describe in Chapter 3, the bodily aspect of the relational schema of being with the client, which is stored in the implicit memory, is activated in supervision. Helene is with her body (the way of talking, voice, gestures, and physiological responses), revealing her state in the therapy, resulting from the interaction with the client. Because of the physiological synchrony and automatic mimicry, we assume that the therapist's reactions are connected to the client's state; and the supervisor's and fellow supervisee Laura's reactions are connected to Helene's state. The physiological parallel process is evident. Quite intense dysregulated physiological responses from all supervision members might point to some hidden trauma process in this psychotherapy.

The supervisor decides to lead the supervisee to explore her experience with the client.

Supervisor:	*What are you experiencing while you are with the client?*
Supervisee Helene:	*I experience that I am not a good enough therapist. She tells me that she has been getting worse since she has been in therapy.* (pause) *And it is difficult for me to hold boundaries with her.*
Supervisor:	*For example, what kind of a boundary would you like to set?*
Supervisee Helene:	*For instance, she is always five minutes late; I do not respond to that. I just leave it …*
Supervisor:	*You swallow it. Through the oesophagus.*
Supervisee Helene:	*Yes, yes.* (pause). *Next to her, I have to find myself; say to myself I am OK as a therapist; to empower the professional part of myself. She asks me personal things. Only a few of my clients allow themselves to ask me something personal.*
Supervisor:	*What does she ask, specifically?*
Supervisee Helene:	*Where do you go to the seaside? How long are you staying there? I think she wants to redirect the focus away from psychotherapy work and her vulnerability.*

The supervisor is aware that the supervision process is also going away from Helene and from the contact with Helene's body. Analysing the client is safer; it may be a distraction and protection from Helene's internal process. Is the supervisor with questions about client Angela "protecting" Helene, leading her to distance herself from her feelings? That may be a parallel process, too. The supervisor decides to provide structure and meaning to what has been said and then to gently bring the supervisee back to mindful awareness of her body.

Supervisor:	*Yes. Let me summarise how I see the case. One thing is that the client wants to be too homely, and she is going away from herself; and for you, it is difficult to set the boundary. The other thing is, connected to the first one: your body started to tremble when you talked about your client. When you reflected on the meaning, you*

*said the client's body shakes, her body is not regulated, and we
can hypothesise that she is traumatised.*

*Your body is a connecting link between therapy and supervision.
From looking at your body in supervision, we can assume how it is
with your body in therapy. As you have difficulties setting
boundaries on the psychological and behavioural level, it may
also be difficult to set boundaries on the body level, and you are
affected by the client's trauma more than necessary.*

Helene and Laura are both nodding.

Supervisor:	*If you agree, let's continue with mindful awareness of our bodies. Later we can cognitively discuss what can be done in therapy.*
Supervisee Helene:	*Now, my body has calmed down. I calmed down when we verbalised that she wanted to be too homely. Earlier I felt trembling and that I was not giving her enough; but when we came to boundaries, and I realised she wanted to be homely, my body calmed down.*

Although on the surface, it looks as if this insight has let the supervisee
calm down, the supervisor feels uneasy with tension in her body, especially
her chest. She hypothesises that the supervision field is not regulated yet and
that the supervisee, by saying she is calm, is not in contact with herself, and
that she may be protecting herself from something painful. This may indicate
a parallel process. The client may behave and protect herself in psychotherapy in a similar way.

Thoughts and questions go through the supervisor's mind: "This is the
calm before the storm; what is it behind this?" She inquires further; she wants
to lead the supervisee to full awareness of her body, the contact, and the
regulation. First, she acknowledges the function of insight.

Supervisor:	*This insight helped you.*
Supervisee Helene:	*Yes. Set the boundaries, set the boundaries.* (pause) *Now I don't feel any trembling. Now I have this revelation- how to go further with her.*

The supervisor still feels uneasiness in her body and wants to connect the
supervisee with her body.

Supervisor:	*OK, you do not feel any trembling; can you tell us what you feel? And Laura and I will also look at our body sensations.*

Supervisee Helene:	(Silence.) *I feel there is some wound in the depth of my chest. Somewhere deep.*
Supervisor and Laura:	(Nodding with compassion)
Supervisee Helene (The pace is slow):	*Yes, somewhere very, very deep ... You mentioned trauma ... yes, I think it is something about that.*

Helene's eyes are moving left and right, and looking up. It looks as if she is processing something.

Supervisee Helene: *Now it is coming more to the surface, what is deep inside; this I feel more and more; it is coming slowly up through my oesophagus, it is scratching. As if I should vomit something up. Yes, it is like that* (showing disgust on her face): *some trauma. Something is in my body that I cannot digest.*

Silence; Helene's eyes moving.

Supervisee Helene:	*And now I am feeling giddy. I have started to sweat.*
Supervisor and Laura:	Nodding.
Supervisee Helene:	*My legs are cold. And it's like I cannot breathe.*

These can be signs of dysregulation and dissociation. Something in Helene, triggered by the psychotherapy session with the client Angela, cannot be digested. It may be that the client's trauma has touched something unprocessed in the psychotherapist Helene, or that Helene synchronised strongly with Angela's dysregulated physiology, or both. The supervisor decides that regulation in supervision is needed. In parallel, the supervision process shows that regulation in psychotherapy sessions is also necessary.

Supervisor:	(Puts her hand on her chest, exhaling deeply.)
Supervisee Laura:	*I also feel immense pressure* (indicating her chest). *It is like when you are holding your breath and have anxiety, which presses on you.*
Supervisor:	*Yes* (still holding her hand on her chest). *What would your body need now?*

With this question, the supervisor wants to activate embodied resources and encourage physiological regulation.

Supervisee Helene:	*Some kind of activity, something physical.*
Supervisor:	*What would you like to do now, at this moment?*

Supervisee Helene: *Now it would suit me to breathe with full lungs.* (Supervisor and Laura both nodding, present); *to stretch and open my chest. Cause I feel that I can't, that everything is squeezing me.*

Supervisor: *Can you do that?*

Supervisee Helene: *Yes.*

Supervisor: *Let's all do that! In our own way. I feel like standing up now.*

The supervisor is feeling pressure in her chest, arms, and legs, so she wants to relax the tension, and regulate herself, too.

Supervisee Helene: *Good idea.*

All three stand. Laura moves her body from the waist from side to side, Helene stretches her hands and chest, and the supervisor shakes her hands. All three of them take their time with their body movements. The movements lead them to regulation and empower their bodies. After some time, they sit down.

When the supervisor feels relieved, lighter, and regulated, she asks:

Supervisor: *What are you feeling now?*

Supervisee Helene: *Now, like new, healthy energy came into my body.*

Supervisor: *Laura?*

Supervisee Laura: *I also feel better after that.*

Supervisor: *Helene, if you think about yourself at the next psychotherapy session: how can you be with your client and at the same time setting a boundary?* (showing with her hand a line in front of her).

The supervisor now returns to the supervisee's initial problem. She wants to connect Helene's new resourceful, regulated body-safe state with the unsafe condition triggered by the therapy with Angela. With this, she wants to encourage memory reconsolidation and transformation of the therapist's relational schema of being with the client (for a theoretical explanation of schema transformation, see Chapter 3).

Supervisee Helene: *I feel myself as a strong pillar, and I say to myself: I am here, this is me, and what I feel from her, that is hers. And that I stay I; I the way I am.* (pause) *If this works, I'll be OK also after the session.*

We can see that the supervisee feels grounded and regulated. Helene found an anchor in herself, which she will take to the next psychotherapy session.

With this resourceful inner state, she will take care of herself and be able to differentiate herself and set boundaries with her client. She will have the capacity to track her own body during the therapy session and the strength to regulate herself and the client in psychotherapy.

Supervisee Helene:　*I also realise I have to be even more aware of my body during therapy. I really see now how psychotherapy influences me on a bodily level.*

Later in the session, the supervisor and supervisees reflect on the supervision session's processes and their meaning for psychotherapy. Based on these insights, they discuss how to lead the psychotherapy with the client further. In the end, they again stressed the importance of the therapist Helene being continually aware of her body in the session and her need for regulation.

Note

1　Adapted from *Integrative psychotherapy: A mindfulness- and compassion-oriented approach* (pp. 145–146), by G. Žvelc & M. Žvelc, 2021, Routledge. Copyright 2021 by G. Žvelc & M. Žvelc. Adapted with permission of the authors and the publisher (Taylor & Francis Ltd, www.tandfonline.com).

Chapter 8

Mindful processing in psychotherapy supervision

In this chapter, we present *the mindful processing method,* a structured method for promoting the processing of supervisees' disturbing experiences related to their psychotherapy work. Mindful processing is an intrapsychic method involving structured moments of silence, where supervisees have space to dive deep into their inner experience with mindful awareness. The supervisor's attuned presence is in the background and helps the supervisee to maintain a mindful stance towards their experience. We illustrate the use of this method with two vignettes from our supervision practice.

In the mindful processing method, the supervisor intentionally invites the supervisee to bring mindful awareness to their present emotions and body sensations related to their experience of the client. The supervisee alternates between mindful awareness of experience and sharing their experience with the supervisor. The supervisee is invited to pay attention to their moment-to-moment experience with curiosity and acceptance. Such a stance towards the inner experience promotes the processing and transformation of disturbing experiences. The method can be described as *relational meditation*, as it gives importance to the mindful presence of both the supervisor and the supervisee. The mindful processing method is based on the assumption that "two aware minds are more powerful than only one" (G. Žvelc, 2012, p. 47). With their mindful presence and compassion, the supervisor helps the supervisee to establish a mindful stance towards their inner experience.

In our previous work, we have presented the mindful processing method focused on its use in psychotherapy (G. Žvelc, 2012, 2014; G. Žvelc & Žvelc, 2008, 2009, 2021). The mindful processing method was primarily developed for the processing of the client's unresolved emotions and traumatic experiences; however, it soon became apparent that it can be instrumental in the supervision process for processing the therapist's countertransference responses (G. Žvelc, 2014; G. Žvelc & Žvelc, 2021). Mindfulness by acceptance and awareness of internal experience promotes the processing of emotions, physical sensations, and cognitions. When we embrace our experience with acceptance and openness, our inner experience starts to transform (G. Žvelc & Žvelc, 2021). Present moment awareness, acceptance,

DOI: 10.4324/9781003194118-11

decentred perspective, and self-compassion are the main processes of change that provide transformation and processing of disturbing experiences. Mindful processing activates the brain's innate error detection system and provides new emotional and relational experiences that promote memory reconsolidation of relational schemas (G. Žvelc & Žvelc, 2021).

Mindful processing in supervision is used for the following purposes:

1 Processing the supervisee's experience of being with the client.
2 Transformation of the supervisee's relational schemas of being with the client.
3 Understanding the client and the dynamics of the psychotherapy relationship.

Processing the supervisee's experience of being with the client

Therapists often leave psychotherapy sessions with painful and dysregulated emotions related to their clients. They may feel fear and anxiety for the client, who is in distress and suffering from depression. Sometimes therapists feel angry towards their client who is stuck and unable to change. Some therapists may feel sexual attraction and develop erotic countertransference. Therapists may carry such feelings from psychotherapy sessions into their everyday life and into the next psychotherapy session. Dysregulated emotions can hinder the psychotherapy process. They may impact the quality of the therapist's relationship with the client and their interventions and may manifest in acting out from the side of the therapist. Such dysregulated emotions may also negatively impact the therapist's personal life. They may negatively affect the therapist's interpersonal relations and their health and ultimately lead to burnout. It is vitally important for therapists to have some means of processing and dealing with such emotions.

In this book, we describe how emotional and physiological regulation is an essential function of supervision and we provide examples of how the supervisor helps the supervisee to regulate emotions and physiology. We also describe a variety of relational mindfulness and compassionate interventions that help the supervisee to regulate and process their dysregulated emotions and physiology.

Mindful processing is a method entirely dedicated to processing the therapist's countertransference experience. It differs from other described interventions in that it involves structured repetitive moments of silence dedicated to mindful awareness of the supervisee's inner experience. The supervisor trusts the supervisee's inner wisdom and innate capacity for processing. This means that the supervisor does not have a predetermined goal for the supervisee and is empty of expectations. The supervisor also does not interfere with the supervisee's processing: Their role is to help the supervisee to maintain a mindful stance towards their inner experience.

The mindful processing method helps the supervisee to process the dys-regulated experience from the bottom-up perspective, beginning with fo-cusing on the therapist's bodily sensations related to their experience of being with the client. The method involves a cycle of mindful processing, where two main phases are repeated cyclically: Mindful awareness of inner experience and sharing the experience with the supervisor. During the mindful awareness phase, the supervisee is invited to observe their inner experience mindfully. It involves moments of silence which allow the supervisee to embrace their experience with awareness and acceptance. After a few moments of silence, the supervisee is invited to share their experience with the supervisor. The cycle of mindful awareness and sharing repeats until the supervisee's ex-perience is processed. After mindful processing, supervisees often feel free from disturbing feelings and bodily sensations related to their psychotherapy session and can separate their own experiences from the client's. They feel as if they are unburdened by the complex emotions and sensations related to the psychotherapy process. When they think about their client, they feel more grounded and present. However, countertransference experiences may also be related to the therapist's unresolved personal issues from their past. In this case, the mindful processing method may help the therapist recognise their wounds and become more aware of what they are related to. The supervisor may, in this case, recommend the supervisee personal therapy.

Transformation of the supervisee's relational schemas of being with the client

In Chapter 3, we introduced the mindfulness- and compassion-oriented transformative supervision model, which describes how mindfulness and compassion processes in supervision transform the supervisee's relational schemas of being with the client. The mindful processing method is one of the methods presented in this book that is used for schema transformation. Repeated experiences of being with the client are recorded in the relational schema of being with the client. Such schemas can be activated both in psychotherapy or in supervision. When the therapist talks about their client in supervision, their relational schemas become activated, and they may re-experience their self-state related to the relationship with the client. Activated relational schemas show in emotional and physiological responses that carry important meaning about the supervisee and their relationship with the client.

The mindful processing method intentionally activates the relational schema of being with the client and makes it open for transformation through the memory reconsolidation process. The memory reconsolidation process is the "brain's innate process for fundamentally revising an existing learning and acquired behavioural responses and/or state of mind maintained by that learning" (Ecker, 2015, p. 4). G. Žvelc & Žvelc (2021) propose that the mindful processing method includes all the necessary phases for therapeutic memory reconsolidation as described by Ecker et al. (2012): Accessing sequence, transformative sequence, and verification. The mindful processing method begins with activating the relational schema of being with the client, which opens the schema for change and transformation. Through the cycle of mindful processing, the supervisee spontaneously gains new insights and experiences contrary to the original relational schema. Our brain is an error-detecting system that continually attempts to minimise the prediction error (Seth, 2013). During mindful processing, the brain automatically detects knowledge contrary to the truth of the original relational schema (G. Žvelc & Žvelc, 2021). When we observe the activation of relational schema from a decentred perspective, we spontaneously become aware of experiences opposing our old truth. The transformation of relational schema occurs when old emotional knowledge is juxtaposed with new disconfirming knowledge (Ecker et al., 2012). The mindful processing method promotes juxtaposition experiences as it invites the supervisee to be mindfully aware at the same time of the original relational schema and new experiences that provide mismatch and experiential disconfirmation. Transformed relational schemas of being with the client positively impact subsequent therapy sessions.

Understanding the client and the dynamics of the psychotherapy relationship

The mindful processing method in supervision also helps raise understanding and insight about the client and the dynamics of the psychotherapy relationship. It can provide valuable insight into the psychotherapy process. In Chapter 3, we discuss how countertransference may carry important information about the client through the process of physiological synchrony. Information about the therapist-client relationship may be embedded in the therapist's subtle bodily sensations, urges, and emotions related to the therapist's experience of the client. Therapists often do not attend to and value these responses and are unaware of their meaning. From our clinical experience, mindful processing sheds light upon subtle somatic countertransference reactions from which meaning can gradually emerge. Mindful awareness of the therapist's somatic experience helps to start the process of subtle understanding of both the client and the therapy process.

Phases of the mindful processing method in supervision

Mindful processing consists of seven phases (G. Žvelc & Žvelc, 2021), which we adapt for the supervision process. The seven phases of mindful processing in supervision are: 1) Preparation, 2) Activation of the relational schema of being with the client, 3) The cycle of mindful processing, 4) Mindful processing of the juxtaposition experiences, 5) Metatherapeutic processing, 6) Reflection on the supervision process, 7) Re-evaluation. Figure 8.1 shows the basic protocol of the mindful processing method.

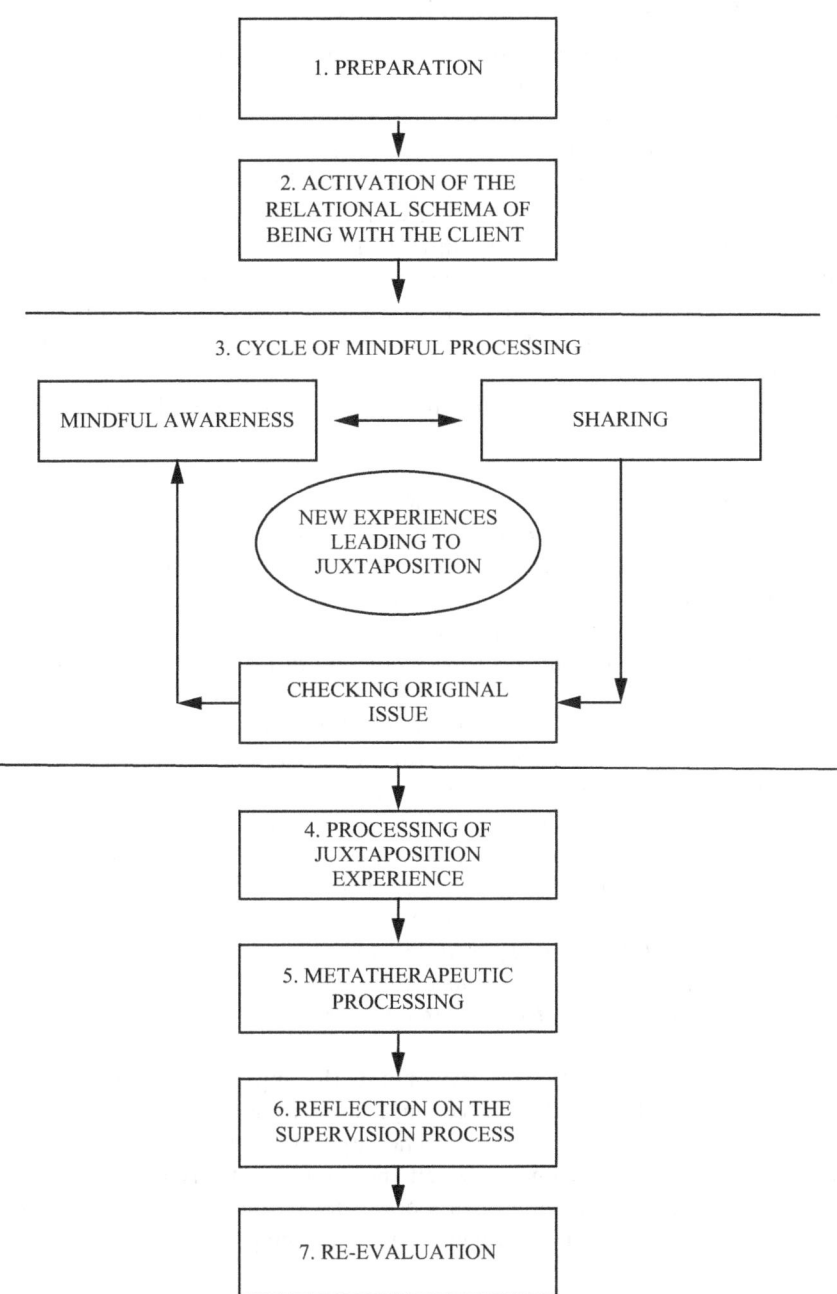

Figure 8.1 The basic protocol of the mindful processing method in supervision.

Note: Adapted from *Integrative Psychotherapy: A Mindfulness- and Compassion-Oriented Approach* (p. 184), by G. Žvelc & M. Žvelc, 2021, Routledge. Copyright 2021 by G. Žvelc & M. Žvelc. Adapted with permission of the authors and the publisher (Taylor & Francis Ltd, www.tandfonline.com).

Phase 1: Preparation

The first phase of mindful processing in supervision involves the contract with the supervisee for mindful processing work and psychological preparation of the supervisor and supervisee. We use mindful processing primarily for the processing of the supervisee's countertransference, which may help them to process dysregulated emotions and body sensations, transform relational schemas of being with the client or gain insight into the psychotherapy process. If the countertransference issues of the supervisee are in the foreground of the supervision, the supervisor may decide to use mindful processing. This involves describing the mindful processing method and then reaching a mutual agreement between the supervisor and supervisee about its use.

The supervisor may introduce mindful processing with the following words:

> "*I will invite you to focus on the body sensations that you experience when you think about your client. Your task is to observe what is happening inside. Gently notice what is happening. Thoughts, images, emotions or body sensations may arise. There is no plan for what should happen. The task is to notice and be aware of your experiences. After some time, I will invite you to share with me what has occurred. You will just tell me what you noticed. After that, I will again invite you to observe and notice what is happening for you at that moment. And then again, I will invite you to share your experiences. So we will alternate between your internal process of experiencing and your sharing of that experience.*
>
> *There is no plan for what should happen. The task is just to be mindful and in contact with your inner experience. If at any time you would like to stop this exercise, you just tell me or lift up your hand. How does that sound to you? Are you willing to proceed with this method?*
>
> *During mindful processing, you can have your eyes closed or focused on something in the room. Do you have any preference? During the session, you can experiment with what feels better for you*".[1]

Before starting, both the supervisor and the supervisee must be psychologically prepared for mindful processing, as the mindful capacity of both the supervisor and supervisee is crucial. The supervisee may experience difficult emotions related to their client, which they may try to avoid and have difficulty experiencing. The supervisor's mindful presence acts as a catalyst for the supervisee's mindful awareness and may help the supervisee accept unpleasant emotional experiences.

The supervisor and supervisee may prepare for mindful processing with brief mindfulness exercises, such as body awareness, breathing, or exercises that promote contact with the observing self. Exercises that promote self-compassion are also helpful, such as the loving hand. The supervisor may do these exercises alongside the supervisee; if the supervision is in the group context, the whole group is invited to participate. It is important that the supervisor and supervisees have the intention to be fully present during mindful processing. The ongoing practice of mindfulness and self-compassion of the supervisor and supervisee is also essential for developing mindful capacity.

Most of our advanced supervisees have a good ability to be mindfully present. However, some less experienced supervisees have difficulty attending to their inner experiences, which may be related to their unresolved personal issues and lack of experience in mindfulness. This is especially the case with unresolved traumatic experiences of the supervisees, which may prevent them from staying within the window of tolerance (D. J. Siegel, 1999) when attending to painful emotions. The supervisor must assess the supervisee's ability to stay present with unpleasant emotions and their readiness to proceed with mindful processing.

For supervisees, who have difficulties staying present during mindful processing, we may introduce the additional focus of attention, such as attention to breathing or any other focus that helps the supervisee to stay present. During mindful processing, such additional focus of attention promotes a decentred perspective and contact with the present moment.

Besides assessing mindful capacity, a good supervisory alliance must also have been established between the supervisor, supervisee, and group members. Sufficient trust and safety are needed so supervisees can feel free to experience and share their inner world with the supervisor.

The preparation phase enables both the supervisor and supervisee to begin the mindful processing method from the position of a loving witness (G. Žvelc & Žvelc, 2021).

Phase 2: Activation of the relational schema of being with the client

In phase 2, we invite the supervisee to activate the relational schema of being with the client.

Awareness of body sensation related to the experience of being with the client

We start mindful processing with the supervisee's awareness of the body-felt experience when they think about psychotherapy with a specific client. This activates the relational schema of being with the client and focuses the supervisee's awareness on their implicit felt-sense experience.

Supervisor: *When you think about your client, what do you feel in your body now? Where do you feel it in your body?*

Sometimes some specific issue related to the client is the source of unpleasant emotions or body sensations, so the supervisor focuses the attention of the supervisee on the specific detail or situation.

"When you think about the client criticising you for not being a good therapist, what do you feel in your body?"

Sometimes the goal of supervision is a better understanding of the client's inner experience. In this case, the supervisee is invited to 'become' the client – to imagine they are their client.

"Imagine that you are your client. Go into the same posture as your client and say some things your client might say ..."

When the supervisee gets into the role of their client, the supervisor invites them to become aware of their body-felt experience:

"What do you feel now in your body? Where do you feel it?"

Utilising the Scale of Physiological Arousal (SPA)

We may use the *Scale of Physiological Arousal* (SPA) to assess the state of physiological arousal related to the supervisee's experience of the client (see Chapter 4, Figure 4.1).

Supervisor: *When you think about your client now, how would you assess your arousal on a scale from −5 to +5. −5 is the most frozen or collapsed you have ever felt, 0 is optimal arousal, and +5 is the most upset and disturbed you have ever felt in your life.*

Focusing on body sensation related to the experience of their client

After the supervisee locates the body sensation and assesses their arousal, we invite them to focus on the body sensation and mindfully observe their experience.

Supervisor: *Focus on that body sensation and just observe what is happening.*

After a few moments, we invite the supervisee to share their experience.

Supervisor: *What is happening now?* or *What are you noticing?*

The supervisee shares their experience with the supervisor.

Phase 2 helps the supervisee to become mindfully aware of the activation of the relational schema of being with the client. In the next phase, they are invited to start the cycle of mindful processing, which is at the heart of the mindful processing method.

Phase 3: Cycle of mindful processing

The cycle of mindful processing involves two main subphases: 1) The supervisee's mindful awareness of internal experience and 2) Sharing with the supervisor. In the cycle, the supervisee alternates between mindful awareness of internal processes and sharing their experience with the supervisor. The cycle of mindful processing also includes checking the original issue.

Subphase 3.1: Mindful awareness of internal experience

The supervisor invites the supervisee to mindful awareness with an invitation to become aware and observe their inner world.

"Be aware of that and notice what is happening inside you".

"Just observe that (sensation, thought, feeling)".

In this subphase, the supervisee is focused on their inner world and becomes aware of their emotions, sensations, and thoughts related to the client's experience. The relational schema of being with the client is activated, and the supervisee mindfully observes their experience. Supervisees may have their eyes open, closed, or focused on a certain point in the room (G. Žvelc & Žvelc, 2021).

During this subphase of mindful awareness, the supervisor makes silent space for the supervisee to immerse in their experience and may occasionally remind the supervisee to maintain mindful awareness with short phrases: *"Just observe that."*, *"Just follow the experience, it is OK whatever comes."*, and *"Make room for this experience".*

Subphase 3.2: Sharing with the supervisor

The supervisor invites the supervisee to share their inner experience.

Tell me what is happening now".

or

"What do you notice?"

The supervisee verbalises their inner experience. The supervisor, with their nonverbal communication, encourages the supervisee to relate to their experience in the present moment, with acceptance and decentred perspective and compassion.

It is important to note that the previous subphase relating to mindful awareness lasts only for about 10–20 seconds. The logic behind this is that the supervisee is attentive to their moment-to-moment experience and shares it with the supervisor. Attunement to the rhythm of the supervisee's processing helps to determine when to invite the supervisee to share. Most supervisees gradually find their natural rhythm regarding mindful awareness and sharing.

If the supervisee can maintain the position of a loving witness and be present with their experience, the supervisor does not interfere with their process. However, if the supervisee starts losing the witnessing position, the supervisor intervenes more actively. For example, if the supervisee becomes distant in relation to their experience, the supervisor invites them to awareness of the present moment and acceptance of experience: *"Just focus on that sensation/emotion."*, *"Make room for this sadness"*. Acceptance can also be promoted by validation: *"This is an important feeling. Just allow yourself to feel it"*.

The invitation to attend to their body sensation also helps the supervisee to come back to the present moment: *"What is happening in your body now?"* Body sensations are like an anchor to which we regularly invite the supervisee to return. This is especially important if supervisees start to intellectualise during mindful processing. Attending to body sensations puts them back on track and in contact with their experiences.

If the supervisee is losing their decentred perspective and becoming merged with their experience, the supervisor invites the supervisee to decentre from their experience and to develop an appropriate distance from their experience: *"Make space between you and your anxiety and observe."*, *"Imagine these disturbing thoughts like leaves in the river that come and go. You are just observing them"*.

We may invite the supervisee into contact with the observing self as this also promotes decentring: *"Imagine that you are there in the room with you and your client, and you are just observing both you and the client. You can observe this from different angles"*.

If the supervisee is merged with the client, it may help if the supervisee imagines they are on one side of the river and on the other side of the river themself and the client:

"Imagine that you are on one side of the river, and on the other side is yourself and your client having psychotherapy. Just observe, listen and look from this side of the river what is happening there".

The position of the loving witness can also be lost if the supervisee becomes judgmental towards themselves. In this case, an invitation to self-compassion may help: "*Imagine yourself in the room with the client and your expression on your face. What do you feel when you see your suffering?*"

If the supervisee starts to become dysregulated and has difficulties staying in the window of tolerance, we provide necessary self-regulation that helps the supervisee regulate their autonomic nervous system (see Chapter 9).

Subphase 3.3: Alternating between mindful awareness and sharing

In mindful processing, the supervisee alternates between mindful awareness and sharing the experience with their supervisor. This alternation happens quite quickly, as the goal is that the supervisee is mindfully aware of their experience moment-by-moment. The supervisor is rhythmically attuned to the supervisee and helps to find the right balance between mindful experiencing and sharing. We usually invite the supervisee to attend to their inner world with mindful awareness for about 10–20 seconds. However, each supervisee processes differently, so some will need more time to come into contact with themselves. For supervisees who have difficulties maintaining mindful awareness, just a few seconds of attention to their inner world may be enough. They may also need more time to share their experience. However, for some supervisees who tend to intellectualise, periods of sharing that are too long may interrupt the contact with their emotions and physical sensations. They may need more prolonged periods of mindful awareness and shorter periods of sharing.

Subphase 3.4: Checking the supervisee's experience of the client

During processing, new insights, images or emotional experiences arise. If the supervisee has achieved significant insight, a shift in perspective or a transformed emotional/body experience, we may invite the supervisee to check their experience of the client again, which re-activates the relational schema of being with the client.

Supervisor: If you think now about your client, what comes up?

We may also invite the supervisee to check their experience of the client if the supervisee's associations are too distant and it seems that the supervisee is not in contact with the main issue. Bringing attention back to the supervisee's experience of the client may re-activate the relational schema of being with the client, and the supervisee may continue the processing.

If the processing is not complete and the supervisee still experiences dysregulated emotions, we invite the supervisee to enter another cycle of processing. If the supervisee reports new insights, changed perspective, and calmness in the body, we may ask the supervisee to check the state of their arousal with the Scale of Physiological Arousal (SPA):

Supervisor: *When you think about the original issue now, how would you assess your arousal on a scale from −5 to +5?*

Phase 4: Mindful processing of the juxtaposition experiences

The supervisee may, during mindful processing, experience new insights and experiences that are contrary to the original relational schema of being with the client. When we invite the supervisee to think again about the client, the relational schema of being with the client is re-activated in the presence of new cognitive, emotional, and physiological experiences. This creates an opportunity for memory reconsolidation and transformation of the relational schema. The supervisee may experience a juxtaposition between new experiences and the original relational schema of being with the client. Such juxtaposition may provide memory reconsolidation and transformation of the relational schema of being with the client. Ecker et al. (2012) describe how repeated juxtapositions between old and new learning may promote memory reconsolidation and transformation of the schemas (Ecker et al., 2012). In this phase, we may intentionally promote explicit awareness of the juxtaposition between old and new learning.

Subphase 4.1: Highlighting the new learning

We may ask the supervisee about new emotional learning and new insights:

"When you think about your client, what is new? How do you feel that in your body?"

Subphase 4.2: Mindful processing of the juxtaposition between old and new learning

In this subphase, we invite the supervisee to be mindfully aware of the contrast between old and new learning, which is crucial for memory reconsolidation (Ecker et al., 2012).

Supervisor: *You felt before that you are bad therapist, but now you experience a feeling of compassion for yourself and a sense that you are OK and you don't have to be perfect. Become aware of the contrast between these two experiences. When you think about both issues together, what do you feel now in your body? Focus on that.*

After this, we initiate another cycle of mindful processing, involving subphase 3.3 related to mindful awareness and sharing of experience. This brings additional integration and transformation of relational schemas.

Phase 5: Metatherapeutic processing

The mindful processing method includes the phase of metatherapeutic processing, initially developed by Diana Fosha. It involves processing the client's or supervisee's experience of positive affect connected to successful psychotherapy work or supervision (Fosha, 2000b, 2000a; Fosha & Conceição, 2019; Fosha et al., 2019; Prenn & Fosha, 2017). If the supervisee experienced a positive, transformational emotional change, we might invite them to process those experiences.

Supervisor: *What is it like for you to have this experience? (name the positive, transformational experience of the supervisee)*

or

Supervisor: *What is it like for you to experience this whole process with me/ the supervision group?*

The supervisor or group members also disclose their own experience of the supervisee's mindful processing, which encourages the supervisee to share their relationship experience.

When the supervisee shares their experience, we may invite them to mindful processing of their transformed emotions (subphase 3.3), which involves cycles of mindful awareness and sharing with the supervisor. Processing positive affect may lead to the experience of wisdom, compassion, self-compassion, flow, and clarity (Fosha et al., 2019), qualities related to the observing/transcendent self.

Phase 6: Reflection on the supervision process

This phase aims to provide closure for mindful processing and integration of the new experience through cognitive processing (G. Žvelc & Žvelc, 2021). The supervisee is invited to reflect upon their experience of mindful processing. The supervisee makes meaning regarding their counter-transference experience, understanding of the client, and the therapeutic process.

The supervisor may also invite the supervisee to pay attention to their countertransference experience during the next psychotherapy session and to use their insights and understanding in psychotherapy with the client.

Phase 7: Re-evaluation

At the next supervision session, we may re-evaluate the processing and check how the supervisee experienced their client in the psychotherapy sessions following the supervision. Supervisees often experience the client in a new way and feel they better understand their client and the psychotherapy process. They come to the following psychotherapy session with regulated emotions, which influences the client positively. Relational schemas of being with the client are often transformed. The processing of their countertransference experiences gives the supervisee more flexibility in psychotherapy and positively impacts both the therapist's interventions and the therapeutic relationship itself.

If the supervisee is still disturbed by countertransference issues, we may continue with mindful processing or use other methods, such as self-compassionate processing (see Chapter 10). In the case of unresolved personal experiences from the therapist's past, additional personal therapy of the supervisee may be advised.

While we present these phases in linear order, they may be creatively used based on the needs of the supervision process. Some phases may even be omitted if other supervision tasks are more pressing or there is a lack of time to proceed with the entire protocol. However, phases 2 and 3, related to the activation of relational schema and the cycle of mindful processing, are essential for the mindful processing method. In the following part of the chapter, we present two vignettes that illustrate the mindful processing method in supervision practice.

Vignette 1: Letting go of an excessive need to rescue the client

The supervisee Sophia felt towards the client an excessive need to rescue him. The client wanted to please his girlfriend, who wanted to have a baby by in vitro fertilisation (IVF). The client was not sure if he wanted to have a baby. The supervisee was overwhelmed with feelings of protection for the client who might be making a serious mistake in his life. In supervision, she recognised that she was overprotective and had difficulties seeing him as autonomous. Even though she had this insight, she still felt the need to rescue him. Because of this, we decided to proceed with mindful processing of her countertransference. We first made a process contract regarding mindful processing and then moved to phase 2, which activates the relational schema of being with the client.

Supervisor: *When you think about this client, what do you feel in your body now?*

Supervisee: *I feel a sense of weight and being trapped in the upper side of the body. Like I am suffocating.*

The activated relational schema shows in unpleasant body sensations of weight in the upper body and suffocation. As the relational schema is now activated, the supervisor moves to phase 3: The cycle of mindful processing.

Phase 3: Cycle of mindful processing

Supervisor:	*Allow yourself to feel that and observe what is happening inside.*
Supervisee:	(mindful awareness)
Supervisor:	What comes up?
Supervisee:	I see him as a small, helpless baby. I feel care towards him.
Supervisor:	Be aware of that small baby and the sense of care.
Supervisee:	(mindful awareness) *I have a need to protect him so that he will not ruin his life.*

The supervisee seems merged with feelings of protection, which is why the supervisor invites the supervisee to decentre from these feelings.

Supervisor:	*Observe the need to protect and the thought "he will ruin his life".*
Supervisee:	(mindful awareness)
Supervisor:	*What is happening now?*
Supervisee:	*I feel like I need to do something – as a rescuer and at the same time there emerged this sense that it is his life and that it is his decision. He has to decide by himself. I have to allow him to decide for himself.*
Supervisor:	*Observe that.*
Supervisee:	(mindful awareness) *The part that feels strongly about rescuing him is getting smaller, and the other part is getting bigger.*
Supervisor:	*What would that part say to the part that wants to rescue him?*

As there are two different self-states, the supervisor invites the supervisee to commence internal communication between the two parts, which may help in the integration process. This is not part of the basic protocol; however, mindful processing is a flexible method that may use different techniques that help the supervisee to process and transform their experience. Working with self-states is one of the ways that may facilitate internal integration and processing.

Supervisee:	(mindful awareness) *There are no words. It is enough that it feels held by the part that is not taking responsibility for the decisions of others.*

As two contradictory parts emerged, which contain two different truths, the supervisor invites the supervisee towards mindful processing of the juxtaposition experience – phase 4.

Phase 4: Mindful processing of juxtaposition experiences

Supervisor:	*It seems that there are two parts. One who feels too much responsibility for the decisions of the client (makes a gesture like*

> *this part is in one hand) and another part who feels that the client is autonomous and can make decisions for themselves (makes a gesture like this part is in the other hand). Become aware of both parts together at the same time.*

Supervisee: (mindful awareness) *They came together. The responsible part is smaller, it is still there, as it is OK that it is in a smaller amount there. The other part is bigger.*

Supervisor: Just stay with that and observe.

Supervisee: (mindful awareness) *I see a flower – they came together and formed a flower. A beautiful image.*

Supervisor: *Just take time and stay with that.*

Supervisee: (mindful awareness) *It is fine. I feel fine.*

It seems that the supervisee can integrate both truths and feels more at peace. Because of that the supervisor invites the supervisee to contact her experience of the client again – Subphase 3.4 Checking the supervisee's experience of the client.

Supervisor: *Think again about your client. What comes up now?*

Supervisee: (mindful awareness) *I still feel care and at the same time that I need to let go of my need to control.*

Supervisor: *Observe that.*

Supervisee: (mindful awareness) *I feel I can let him make his own decision. I don't see that as a catastrophe anymore. He will have to bear the consequences of his decisions. I feel fine now.*

Through mindful processing of the excessive need to rescue the client there emerged another truth – that other people are autonomous. While the supervisee already had a cognitive insight about that, she experienced it on a deeper emotional level after mindful processing. As the supervisee's emotional experience was transformed, the remaining part of the supervision involved metatherapeutic processing (phase 5) and reflection on the supervision process (phase 6).

Mindful processing helped the supervisee integrate both perspectives – the importance of care for the client and seeing the client as autonomous with his responsibility. Most importantly, the supervisee did not feel trapped anymore and felt a lesser need to take an inappropriate amount of responsibility in the following sessions with the client. This also helped her work with the client towards setting more appropriate boundaries between himself and his girlfriend, as the client was preoccupied with pleasing her. The supervisee's original relational schema of being with the client was related to taking too much responsibility towards another person. Through mindful processing, the schema was transformed towards a more balanced view of appropriate care and seeing another person as autonomous. This influenced subsequent psychotherapy sessions with the client.

Vignette 2: From helplessness to strength and insight

The supervisee, Petra, described a sense of helplessness related to the client. She felt overwhelmed, helpless, and "sucked" into the client's story. These feelings stayed with her after the end of the psychotherapy sessions and even at home. She described how her client found out that his wife was having personal and intimate discussions with another man. The client was very upset and angry with fantasies of killing the man. He was self-medicating by drinking alcohol.

The supervisor and supervisee made a contract about using the method of mindful processing as the supervisee's countertransference negatively impacted her work with the client (phase 1 of mindful processing). As the supervisee was already quite versed with the mindful processing method, no additional preparation phase was necessary. The supervision took place in a group of three supervisees.

The supervisor first invites Petra to become aware of the body sensation related to the experience of being with the client. This activates her relational schema of being with the client (phase 2 of mindful processing).

Phase 2: Activation of the relational schema of being with the client

Supervisor: *When you think about this client, what do you feel in your body now?*

Supervisee: *I feel a sense of tension in the neck, a very uncomfortable feeling.*

Supervisor: *Focus on that tension in the neck and observe with curiosity what is happening.*

Supervisee: (mindful awareness)

Supervisor: *What comes up?*

Supervisee: *Now I feel a sense of confusion, helplessness … like being in a fog.*

After focusing on the body sensation, the supervisee experiences a sense of being in a fog, which may be a sign of hypoarousal of the autonomic nervous system. As the supervisor knows that the supervisee can regulate herself with mindful awareness, he proceeds with the next phase – the cycle of mindful processing (phase 3).

Phase 3: The cycle of mindful processing

Supervisor: *Mm-hm. Observe and be curious.*

Supervisee: (mindful awareness) *Now comes an image of having a rope around my neck. It is very painful.*

The image of having a rope around her neck brings intense feelings.

Supervisor: *Just breathe in and out of that feeling.*

As the supervisor senses that the supervisee is dysregulated, he proposes that she starts to breathe in and out of that feeling. Breathing may provide regulation of physiological and emotional arousal, which helps the supervisee to stay in the optimal arousal zone and process emotions.

Supervisee: (mindful awareness)
Supervisor: *What is happening now?*
Supervisee: *No, not that!! I do not want that. (with a powerful, angry voice and strength).*

The supervisee looks and sounds angry.

Supervisor: *Allow yourself to feel that "No!"*
Supervisee*:*   (mindful awareness) *Now I am giving away that rope. And the rope has fallen to the ground.*
Supervisor: *Allow yourself to be with whatever comes.*
Supervisee: (mindful awareness) *Now it is calming down.*

After experiencing anger, the supervisee starts to calm down, which is visible in her posture and her tone of voice.

Supervisor: *Just feel this calming down.*
Supervisee: (mindful awareness) *Sense of being calm … Now it is OK. I have a sense that I am here and the client is there.*

The supervisee feels more regulated and has a greater sense of separation between herself and the client.

Supervisor: *Just take time and stay in touch with that.*
Supervisee: *It is fine. I am OK.*

The supervisee experiences a transformation of emotion from feeling helpless and confused to feeling angry and eventually to a safe state of calmness. As her feelings are transformed and regulated, the supervisor invites the supervisee to contact her experience of the client again (subphase 3.4 Checking the supervisee's experience of the client).

Supervisor: *Now, think again about your client. What comes up?*
Supervisee: (mindful awareness) *He is really in danger. Maybe he is feeling suicidal. He is feeling helpless.*

Mindful processing brings insight into the client's state of mind and helps with understanding the client.

Supervisor: Just observe that.
Supervisee: (mindful awareness) *I am feeling OK like I don't carry that anymore. I feel more separation between myself and him.*
Supervisor: Just observe that.
Supervisee: (mindful awareness) *I have never thought that I would hang myself – that's not mine. It is not congruent with my general mood. I see that he is really in terrible pain.*

The relational schema of being with the client is transformed. The supervisee experiences a greater separation between herself and the client, and her emotions are not overwhelming as they were at the beginning of the supervision session. Her perception of the client changed. When she described the client at the beginning of the session, she seemed bothered by the client's anger and aggressive fantasies. Now she understands that there is helplessness or even suicidal ideation behind the client's anger and rage. As the supervisee experienced intense emotions during mindful processing, we take time to process her experience in the group (phase 5 – metatherapeutic processing). Both supervisor and other members of the group share their experiences related to the process. They were all impacted by the intensity of the supervisee's feelings and touched by the shift in the supervisee's experience.

After metatherapeutic processing, we invite the supervisee to reflect on the supervision process (phase 6).

Supervisor: When you think about this process, how would you connect it to the psychotherapy session?
Supervisee: I feel now calmer and have a sense of greater strength. By being fully aware of the feeling, it's helped me to find strength. Probably I identified with his helplessness, and now I feel a greater boundary between him and myself. I also see that behind his anger, there is great pain. I will also deal with possible suicidal ideation next time in the therapy.

In this example, the supervisee was merged with her countertransference at the beginning of the supervision session. Mindful processing helped her to process her dysregulated physiology and emotions, which transformed into calmness, a sense of strength, and a greater boundary between herself and the client. The original relational schema of being with the client was transformed. This helped her to come to the next psychotherapy session with a different state of mind. She felt more grounded and in contact with herself. Her arousal level was within the window of tolerance. This helped her to deal more effectively with a difficult client situation. Mindful processing also brought her insight into the client. She hypothesised that behind the client's rage was an enormous pain and even possible suicidal ideation.

Note

1   Adapted from *Integrative psychotherapy: A mindfulness- and compassion-oriented approach* (p. 187), by G. Žvelc & M. Žvelc, 2021, Routledge. Copyright 2021 by G. Žvelc & M. Žvelc. Adapted with permission of the authors and the publisher (Taylor & Francis Ltd, www.tandfonline.com).

Chapter 9

Methods of emotional and physiological regulation in supervision

This chapter provides clinical applications of the construct of emotional and physiological regulation in supervision. We present the Triple R model of the supervisor's tasks and interventions for emotional and physiological regulation. In two vignettes, we illustrate how dysregulation in psychotherapy is, through a parallel process, relived in supervision and convey how the supervisor can lead the process towards regulating the supervision field, which will influence the psychotherapy field.

The Triple R model describes three main supervision tasks related to emotional and physiological regulation in supervision: 1) Recognition of emotional and physiological dysregulation, 2) Regulation of physiology and emotions, and 3) Reflection on the meaning of dysregulation (Figure 9.1).

Recognition of emotional or physiological dysregulation through mindful body awareness

The first essential supervision task is being aware of physiological processes in the here and now and recognising dysregulation of the supervision field. This means detecting if one or more supervision members are becoming emotionally and physiologically hyper- or hypo-aroused. The source of dysregulation may come from any supervision member and, through the process of physiological synchrony, spreads to other members of supervision. Mostly the dysregulation originates from within the supervisee who is presenting the case.

The royal path to recognising dysregulation in supervision is through mindful body awareness. The supervisor and supervisee need to be attentive to their bodies and validate the importance of changes in the body.

To encourage recognition of physiological states, the supervisor uses the following interventions:

a   Mindful awareness of their own body and physiological state.
b   Mindful observation of the supervisee's body.
c   Promoting the supervisee's mindful awareness of their physiological state.

DOI: 10.4324/9781003194118-12

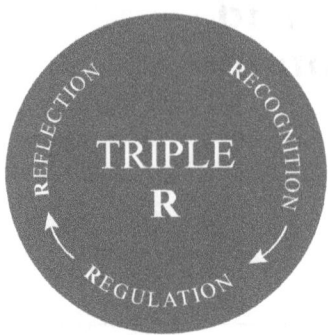

Figure 9.1 Triple R model of emotional and physiological regulation.

The supervisor's primary task is to be mindful of what is happening in their own body during the course of the supervision session, noticing any changes in their physiological processes and evaluating their physiological states. For instance, supervisor Ted becomes mindfully aware of a pervading feeling of restlessness in his body, feels his heart racing, and realises his body is in hyperarousal. Besides acknowledging his hyperarousal, he validates it; he knows these detected changes in his body are significant. Supervisor Ted hypothesises that these perceived body sensations might provide important information about his interaction with the supervisee and probably tell a not yet revealed story of the supervisee's interaction with their client. He also reflects that he may be synchronised with the supervisee's physiology, which gives him a clue that the supervisee is probably also dysregulated. This example shows how mindful awareness is linked to reflection and provides meaning to observed body signs.

The supervisor's next task is to observe the supervisee's body. The supervisor notices changes in the supervisee's body (movements, posture, facial expression, tone of voice, colour of the skin, etc.). The supervisor also observes the bodies of other supervision members. Changes in their bodies are significant. The supervisor wants to detect if dysregulation is taking place.

The next significant supervisor's task is to raise the supervisees' mindful awareness of their physiological state. This requires mindful awareness of the supervisee's body and evaluating their physiological states here and now in the supervision session. The supervisor facilitates the supervisees' interoception by inquiring and acknowledging their body processes.

Contracting for mindful awareness and regulation

To implement mindful awareness and regulation in the supervisory relationship, we need first to inform the supervisee of their significance. Then we contract with them to work on mindful awareness and regulation of physiological states in supervision. In the contract, we agree that when the supervisor or supervisee notices dysregulated physiology and emotions within the supervision session, we will introduce a mindful pause to initiate mindful awareness and regulation. This contracting is very important since it enables the supervisee to willingly interrupt the dysregulation process and make space for mindful observation. Dysregulation has strong inertia; a person in a dysregulated state is likely to be resentful of such a pause, wanting to hold on to this state. When supervisees (supervisors or clients) are hyperaroused, they are urged to talk, explain, and proceed with the content, even though it is unfruitful (dysregulation disables integration). Remembering the contract helps supervisees to comply with the supervisor's suggestion for a mindful pause and are willing to mindfully observe, even though they may not see its usefulness at that moment.

Mindful pauses in supervision

The supervisor initiates a mindful pause in supervision and leads the supervisee to make space for mindful observation of their body (breathing, heartbeat, skin temperature, sensations in different parts of the body, etc.). Usually, we suggest a mindful pause with the following words: "*Teresa* (the name of the supervisee), *are you willing to pause for a moment and be aware of what you are feeling in your body right now? I will do the same and observe my body; and you, Peter and Katarina, if you agree, do the same*". In this way, we invite other group members, if there is group supervision, to be part of the mindful pause.

When the supervisor notices that the supervisee is dysregulated, they need to temporarily put aside cognitive discussion of the case and make space for present moment experience. We have learned that mindful awareness of the body is a very effective way to bring supervisees (and supervisors) into the present moment and into contact with themselves. The supervisees' awareness of their physiological and emotional imbalance comes before other supervision processes. When supervisees become aware of their dysregulation, we can only then explicitly lead them to further regulation and reflection on the meaning of their dysregulated states.

Regulation of physiology and emotions

When we become aware of the emotional and physiological dysregulation of supervision member(s) in the supervision session, we promote regulation. If one member of the supervision is hyper- or hypo-aroused, that influences other supervision members. As supervisors, we want to stop dysfunctional synchrony among members and transform the dysregulated supervision field into a balanced, regulated physiology field. As we explain in Chapter 4, cognitive processes are optimal only when the supervision members' emotions and physiology are regulated. It is only in this state that supervisees are open to learning, and the regulated emotions and physiology of the supervisees are then transmitted back to the psychotherapy relationship.

The supervisor uses two main methods connected to the regulation process:

a Self-regulating.
b Co-regulating the supervisee.

The process when a person regulates themselves is called self-regulation. When one or more people regulate another person(s), this is co-regulation (Porges, 2017) or relational regulation (G. Žvelc & Žvelc, 2021). Relational regulation can run implicitly, without a conscious attempt to regulate another, or explicitly, with an active decision to regulate the other.

The supervisor is the one who is to be attentive to their own and to their supervisee's emotional and physiological states and initiate regulation within themselves and regulation of the supervisee when needed. When the supervisor regulates themselves, they return to the window of tolerance, which enables them to continue leading the supervision efficiently and to co-regulate supervisees. The supervisor regulates the supervisee in two ways: Implicitly and explicitly. The supervisor automatically and implicitly regulates the supervisee when their own autonomic nervous system (ANS) is balanced. The supervisee's physiology synchronises with the supervisor's balanced physiology. Through neuroception (Porges, 2017), the supervisee subconsciously detects the supervisor's safe physiological state (through the supervisor's eyes, facial gestures, body expressions, prosodic voice, etc.), which helps the supervisee's ANS to come into balance. Regulated and secure experiences in supervision are encoded in the supervisee's implicit relational schemas. This implicit memory of safety and regulation is then activated within the therapist in the therapeutic relationship.

Mindfulness as a tool for regulation

The supervisor can also regulate the supervisee in explicit ways. The primary strategy we suggest is encouraging mindfulness processes within the supervisee: Present moment awareness, acceptance, and decentred perspective (G. Žvelc & Žvelc, 2021). Methods of relational mindfulness and compassion (see Chapter 2) promote accepting awareness of emotions and body sensations that spontaneously lead to regulation. This is congruent with research and clinical practice that shows that mindfulness encourages regulation (Farb et al., 2012; Goldin & Gross, 2010; A. M. Hayes & Feldman, 2004; Price & Hooven, 2018; Taren et al., 2013; Teper et al., 2013; Vago & Silbersweig, 2012; G. Žvelc & Žvelc, 2021).

We suggest the supervisor first leads the supervisee to mindful awareness of their body sensations and physiological states. By mindful awareness of their body, the supervisee can come in touch with their needs and adaptive action tendencies (like breathing deeply, moving, etc.). In this way, we encourage the supervisee to use their own body's resources to regulate. If the supervisee is hyperaroused, downregulation and slowing down are needed. We can encourage the supervisee to begin deep, slow breathing, with a longer out-breath than in-breath, feeling their feet on the ground, etc. If the supervise is hypoaroused, then activation, bringing life to their body-mind, is crucial. We encourage the supervisee to move, starting with minor changes and gradually intensifying them. For instance, we can initiate slightly deeper breathing, moving fingers, wrists, and feet. When the supervisee regains some of their safety, we can indicate standing, stretching, moving, shaking, and jumping. We, as supervisors, do that alongside the supervisee; we are modelling, bringing more energy between the two of us, and reducing shame (which is usual within a hypoaroused state). In all of the initiated body changes (like deeper breathing) and body movements (like shaking), we are mindfully aware of the effect of those changes. We present practical examples of physiological regulation in the vignettes.

Promoting compassion and self-compassion as a strategy for regulation

Self-compassion is positively linked to emotional regulation (Barlow et al., 2017; Bates et al., 2021; Diedrich et al., 2016; Finlay-Jones, 2017; Inwood & Ferrari, 2018; Scoglio et al., 2015; Vettese et al., 2011). Bringing a kind, caring, and loving attitude to themselves as a person and as a professional helps supervisees (or supervisors) raise safety in themselves, which is the essential component of regulation. It allows the supervisee to accept themselves as a therapist, complete with their possible shortcomings. The supervisees often doubt their work and criticise themselves (M. Žvelc, 2017). This destabilises their nervous system and leads them to dysregulated states. With the help of self-kindness and self-compassion, they can face and hold difficult feelings, start to accept themselves, the defensive processes back off, and the supervisee resets their safety and returns to an optimal arousal zone.

Difficulties in physiological regulation in supervision

It sometimes happens that the supervision system stays dysregulated at the end of the supervision session. In our experience, different factors may contribute to this, including the supervisor's or supervisee's strong counter-transference, which is often connected to unresolved trauma, a rupture in the supervisory alliance, or the supervisor's or supervisee's current life stress.

Sometimes more space for reflection is needed, and the dysregulation and the rupture can be resolved in the following supervision session, which will bring an opportunity to observe the previous supervision session at a greater distance and to reflect on it. It will be another opportunity for regulation or/ and rupture repair. When supervisees have some unresolved trauma triggered by the therapy with their client or face some demanding life stress, it is necessary to deal with that issue in their personal psychotherapy. We suggest that continuously non-regulated supervision sessions correlate to the supervisee's burnout and may lead to the supervisee dropping out. The supervisor may need to talk to their own supervisor regarding difficulties in supervision. It can happen that a supervisee cannot open the space for mindful awareness of their state in supervision and stays dysregulated. In this case, the supervisor helps the supervisee to become aware of this and to reflect on it. It is not, however, the supervisor's role to do personal therapy with the supervisee. If dysregulation of the supervisee and their incapability of mentalising their physiological state is persistant, then we have a critical event in supervision (Ladany et al., 2005; M. Žvelc, 2017). During the supervision session, the supervisor may reflect on the following questions: "Is there a supervisory alliance rupture, and the supervisee does not feel safe enough to explore their bodily countertransference? Are there some other deficiencies in the supervisee's functioning? Maybe this deficiency is temporary, and additional personal therapy is needed? Or perhaps it shows some more permanent deficits in the supervisee's capacities for therapeutic work".

We would emphasise here that our aim in supervision is not healing the therapist when we provide regulation. As supervisors, we need to be conscious of not taking over the work of other professional fields (like psychotherapy).

Reflecting on the meaning of dysregulation

The third essential supervision process, reflection, is related to exploring the meaning of emotional and physiological processes occurring during the supervision session. We want to understand how and why the supervision members become dysregulated; what is the story behind it?

The supervisor's tasks are:

a   Reflecting on the meaning of their and the supervisee's physiological states.
b   Promoting supervisees' reflection on the meaning of their physiological states.

The supervisor is mindfully aware of their own inner states, primarily their body/physiological state, and recognises hyper- or hypo-arousal within themselves. They need to be curious about the origins of this dysregulation. They may ask themselves: "*How come my breath is shallow, shoulders are tight, and legs are cold, right now, here in the supervision session?*" Such reflective questions cue the supervisor that the supervisee may also be dysregulated. This can mean different things: That the supervisee was dysregulated as a therapist in the therapy session, that there is a rupture in the supervisory alliance or that the supervisee is under intensive stress from other reasons. Sometimes, the supervisor's changes in emotions and physiology may stem from their own internal process, like recalling their own problems and worries during the session. Nevertheless, looking from an intersubjective perspective, their anxious mind and concerns about their issues can be co-constructed by the supervisee's anxious state.

With the help of the supervisor, supervisees can ask themselves and explore: "*What is the meaning of my particular sensation I have in supervision (like having a pain in my chest, pressure in my stomach, heart beating, or other …)? Why do I become hyper- (or hypoaroused) when presenting this case?*"

The supervisee's body in the supervision session is telling a significant story about the supervisee's interaction with their client. While remembering the therapy session with a particular client, the therapist's implicit body-emotional memory related to the relational schema of being with the client is activated. Being attentive to the supervisee's body sensations and physiological states enables the members of supervision to mentalise the meaning of these states. They reveal hidden, unspoken, unconscious aspects of the interaction with the client. Reflection on these states and mentalisation about their meaning leads to new insights regarding the therapist's countertransference, dynamics in the therapeutic relationship, and possibly the client's physiological states and feelings.

Reflection takes the process of regulation in supervision one step further. Regulation is essential for influencing the supervisee's way of being with their client, and reflection helps them to raise further awareness and insight into the psychotherapy process. Both are vital for effective supervision. Reflection can also contribute to regulation (Hill, 2015).

These described processes of mindful body awareness, regulation, and reflection can alternate very quickly; sometimes they are parallel, and sometimes they intertwine. The order can change, but the primary step is always mindful awareness of inner bodily states (within the supervisor and/or the supervisee) and recognition of physiological or emotional dysregulation. Activating the observing self within the supervision members enables them to adopt a decentred position to their experience, become present, accept the experience, and be kind to themselves. All these processes enable physiological and emotional regulation.

The following two vignettes show the practical use of emotional and physiological regulation in supervision. The first vignette shows the regulation of hypoarousal in the supervisee, while the second one presents the regulation of hyperarousal. We invite the reader to connect the presented supervision processes with the supervisor's actions in the vignettes. To make it easier to do this, we remind you about the supervision tasks, methods, and interventions in Table 9.1 below.

Table 9.1 Methods and interventions of the Triple R model

Supervision tasks	Supervisor's methods and interventions
Recognition of emotional and physiological dysregulation	Mindful awareness of their physiological state. Observing the supervisee's body. Promoting the supervisee's mindful awareness of their physiological state.
Regulation of physiology and emotions	Self-regulating. Co-regulating the supervisee.
Reflection on the meaning of dysregulation	Reflecting on the meaning of their own and their supervisee's physiological states. Promoting the supervisee's reflection on the meaning of their physiological states.

Vignette 1: Physiological regulation of hypoarousal in the supervision session

In triadic supervision, the supervisee Monica is presenting a particular case with her client Sonja, who self-injured herself badly.

Supervisee Monica: *Sonja wasn't aware when she cut herself; she just "woke"up and saw the sheets were red with blood.*

When you, the reader, read these lines, what do you feel in your body now? While the supervisee is talking, the supervisor feels her hands are becoming unusually cold, she feels freezing in her legs, and her breath is shallower. She recognises that she is entering the hypoarousal zone of her ANS. The supervisor starts to self-regulate by abdominal breathing and gently moving her hands and legs. She observes the supervisee's body and notices that the hands of the supervisee are pale, and it seems to her that she feels the coldness of the supervisee's hands. On that basis, the supervisor begins to reflect: "*What is the meaning of this? These could be a sign of a hypoarousal of ANS. Is there something happening with the supervisee? Is she freezing? It's possible; she's telling a horrible story about her client. The client was dissociating; is the supervisee dissociating?*"

Supervisor   *While you are talking about your client, what are you*
(asks the supervisee):   *noticing in your body now?*
Supervisor (turns to   *And, you, please, also check what you feel in your*
the other supervisee):   *body.*

The supervisor encourages mindful awareness and recognition of the physiological state within all supervision members, including herself. Dysregulated physiological states through dysfunctional physiological synchrony influence the whole supervision system, and group members can react to it in various ways.

Supervisee Monica:	*Oh, I can hardly feel my hands and legs. I feel like I'm being paralysed. It's quite a scary sensation.*
Supervisor (nods and turns to the other member):	*And you?*
Another supervisee:	*In the beginning, I felt nothing. I am aware that I dissociated and wandered away with my thoughts. Now I am aware of the pressure in my chest.*

Feeling paralysed and hardly sensing her body is a sign of the hypoarousal of the supervisee Monica. The dissociation of the other supervisee is also a sign of dysregulation, probably in the direction of hypoarousal. As you can see, at the beginning of our vignette the supervisor was, through physiological synchronisation, resonating with similar symptoms that supervisees were experiencing; the signs of hypoarousal. Because the supervisees and the supervisor were becoming dysregulated when Monica was talking about her client, there is a high probability that in their therapy Monica as the therapist and her client were dysregulated, too. The body states of the supervisor and the supervisees (cold, freezing hands and legs; difficulties in sensing the body, feeling paralysed, and stopping breathing) were markers for the supervisor to start physiological regulation.

Supervisor: *Mm-hm, mm-hm. These are the feelings that might be connected to therapy with Sonja. Let's breathe … and let's move our hands and legs.*

The supervisor in this intervention first reflects on the supervisees' states and gives some explanation before starting to regulate the supervisees actively. The supervisor also takes deeper breaths and moves her feet, regulating herself. With the description *"These are the feelings that might be connected to therapy with Sonja"*, the supervisor also validates and normalises the supervisee's sensations to help the supervisee find a decentred perspective and not be merged with their feelings. She also lets the supervisee know that these sensations carry meaning. With this, the supervisee can have a sense of greater control.

Both supervisees and the supervisor move their hands and legs. Monica's chest movements are more visible now. The supervisor feels in her body that the movements have helped her a little, but that the energy in her body is still stuck and not yet running freely. She also sees and feels that Monica is also not yet in a balanced state.

Supervisor (to Monica):   Notice ... what would your body like to do now?

The supervisor leads Monica to mindful awareness of her body's adaptive action tendencies. Realising what her body needs will then help Monica to self-regulate.

Supervisee Monica: To stand up ... move.
Supervisor: Sure ... let's do that. Let us all do that!

The supervisor stands next to Monica and suggests the other supervisee does the same. With this, she increases the sense of safety in the group and reduces possible feelings of shame within Monica. A person in hypoarousal often feels threatened by people and is prone to feel high levels of shame. By encouraging the other supervisee to stand and move, the supervisor also helps the group energy level to rise (hypoarousal is the zone with a deficient energy level) and also helps the other supervision member to regulate herself. Their movements gradually intensify; first, they walk around the room, shake their hands, and later jump and smile. Hypoarousal is a survival reaction when detecting a life threat. A person or an animal becomes immobilised, feigning death in order to survive. With breathing and movements, we mobilise the body bringing back energy and life, which counters immobilisation and death (Levine, 1997).

The supervisor feels her energy is returning to her body, her hands and legs are warm, and she breathes freely. She asks the supervisees how they are. Monica feels warmth in her hands and legs and feels alive again. The other supervisee feels her legs steady on the ground; the pressure in her chest has gone, and she is breathing more easily.

Supervisor (suggests   How do you understand what happened?
sitting and then asks the group):   How can we explain the states we were feeling?

She promotes the supervisee's reflection on the meaning of their physiological states.

Supervisee Monica: The client must feel the same ... she was freezing, dissociating while cutting herself.
Supervisor: Yes.
Another supervisee: And, I wonder ... in what states were you and Sonja in the therapy while she was talking about the cutting?
Supervisee Monica: Indeed, yes, I think I just dissociated, went away a few times during the last therapy session. It was too much for me.

After the supervisee, supervisor, and the other group member came back to the window of tolerance, the supervisor initiated the mentalisation process within the supervisees, looking to understand what happened during both the supervision session and the therapy. Based on that, the supervisee gains new insight into how to be in therapy and how to lead it. With arriving at the window of tolerance, the cognitive functions of the members are restored, and only then can they use them optimally, to think and decide non-defensively, flexibly, and creatively.

Later, after the discussion about the meaning and getting new insights, the supervisor asks:

Supervisor: *Monica, when you think about the next therapy session, what happens in your body?*

With this question, we are checking if Monica's previous relational schema of being with her client Sonja has changed, and if it has, we simultaneously elaborate on the change.

Supervisee Monica: *Yeah, it is better now; I feel I am present.*

We can see that Monica's schema of being with her client Sonja has changed significantly. At the beginning of the session, Monica's relational schema of being with the client was related to hypoarosual. Monica felt threatened and was avoiding contact with both herself and the client. Through the process of emotional and physiological regulation, the relational schema of being with the client transformed. Monica was feeling better and present, which is a sign of a balanced physiological response.

Supervisor: *Mm-hm. Do you have any thoughts or insights about the next session?*

Supervisee Monica: *I am going to monitor my body regularly during the therapy … to keep me present, and then regulate myself and the client …, like we did it here.*

Besides the transformation of the relational schema of being with her client, Monica has developed a new relational schema related to the process of emotional and physiological regulation. This was a new skill that she could regularly use in her psychotherapy.

A month later, the supervisee told the supervisor that the most important thing for her was that she regularly monitors her inner states during therapy sessions and promotes regulation. Since then, she reported that she doesn't feel so tired after the therapy sessions as she did before. Supervision work done in this way not only helps therapists to optimise the therapy, but it also helps them take care of themselves and their physical health and optimise their well-being.

Vignette 2: Working with hyperarousal in supervision

In this supervision session, Tanja, the supervisee, says she feels stuck in the therapy with client Simona. The client has been in therapy for three months. The therapist, Tanja, doesn't see any changes or progress in this therapy. The client is emotionally unstable, anxious, and has sleep difficulties; the symptoms have not improved. Tanja has thoughts between sessions that the client is too much for her and privately she hopes that her client won't come back and will leave the therapy. In this supervision session, Tanja would like to know what to do differently for more effective psychotherapy. The supervisor notices that Tanja presents the case in a fast rhythm without taking time to inhale. The supervisor hypothesises that Tanja is physiologically in the hyperarousal zone of her ANS. The supervisor is also aware that while Tanja is talking, she is irritated by the supervisee's way of talking and that her sympathetic nervous system is being activated (faster heartbeat, irregular breathing, restlessness in her body). When she recognises she is becoming hyperactivated, she self-regulates (slower breathing, leaning a little back from the supervisee). She takes a decentred perspective, making space between the supervisee and herself and between her awareness and the content of her experience. She reflects that a parallel process is probably going on. The dysregulated field in the supervision, which is just happening, may parallel a dysregulated therapy process. Client Simona has a more or less constantly dysregulated ANS in her life. She brings this dysregulated state with her into therapy, and the therapist synchronises with the hyperarousal of the client. Tanja gradually formed the relational schema of being with the client Simona, which contains physiological hyperactivation, feeling unsafe and anxious, and a tendency to reject the client. The ongoing dysregulated field in the therapy is the hindering factor in the treatment which Tanja was presenting. It probably contributes to therapy stagnation. The supervisor decides to help Tanja raise mindful body awareness, recognise her physiological state, and to regulate it.

Supervisor:	*Tanja, I would like to ask you to direct your attention to your experience here and now. What are you noticing in your body?*
Supervisee (answers right away):	*Nothing special.*

Tanja did not take time for mindful awareness. Her answer indicates experiential avoidance.

Supervisor: We cannot get in touch with ourselves so quickly. Take your time, breathe, and notice what is happening inside you now.

The supervisor decided to continue with the gentle inquiry about the supervisee's inner state. At the same time, she regulates the supervisee with "permission" to take space and time for her self-observation. The supervisee does not allow herself to breathe and slow down (in supervision and therapy). The supervisor is modelling how to pause and invite mindful awareness to the busy and agitated mind.

Supervisee (after pausing):   *My body is shaking, and I feel pressure in my chest.*

The supervisee is becoming mindfully aware of her inner state here and now.

Supervisee (continues):   *But, you know, I am not like that in the therapy. In therapy, I am ok.*

The supervisee's last statement may indicate that the supervisee feels blamed for feeling this way by the supervisor or herself. It looks as if she feels that her safety in supervision is compromised. The supervisor decides to re-establish the alliance and the feeling of security. She uses a gentle voice and a reassuring look. With this, she conveys safety to the supervisee and co-regulating her. In the subsequent intervention, she facilitates mindful awareness of the supervisee by actively encouraging the decentred position and loving acceptance, which can also evoke self-compassion. With this, she helps the supervisee to stay present.

Supervisor: *I am interested in what it is like for you in therapy with Simona. If you agree, let's turn your attention in a kind, loving way to your body again. Just notice, just observe how your body responds here and now. I will observe mine, as well.*

The supervisor believes that what Tanja feels in psychotherapy may be revealed by exploring Tanja's body sensations here in supervision. Tanja's presentation of psychotherapy with the client activates her implicit relational schema of being with the client. The therapist's body is right now re-membering and telling an important story, the story of how she feels in the session with her client. The supervisor hypothesises that it is a painful story, and that's why Tanja wants to avoid it and try to evade body awareness.

Supervisee (Silence.   *Now the pain is moving to my shoulder. Oh, it's like*
Breathes slowly and   *the pain I've had in the last three months. That*
talks at a slower pace):   *corresponds with the time Simona came into*
therapy. O, shit, do you think it may be connected?

The slower pace of breathing and talking is a sign of self-regulation. The supervisee also reflects on the meaning of her physiological state. Now, with the supervisee more in contact with herself, the supervisor decides to ask her about her experience in therapy.

Supervisor: How do you feel in the therapy session while working with Simona?

Supervisee: I feel ok then.

Silence. It looks as if the supervisee is processing something.

Supervisee (continues): I think I am not really attentive to what I feel then; I want to give all of my attention to Simona. I am very empathic. I am all of me for her there. (Silence) I recall now that I often don't sleep well when I have had a session with Simona.

Tanja is recognising her dysregulation.

Supervisor: In today's supervision, while you were talking about the therapy with Simona, your physiological state changed. When we were observing your state, you noticed that you were agitated. At first, you didn't realise that.

Supervisee: Do you think I can be hyperactivated while I am doing therapy with Simona and not be aware of it?

Supervisor: Yes, I do think so. We can look at what happened during our supervision session through the lens of a parallel process. Here, in the supervision, there was a hyperactivated, dysregulated state that would suggest there is a dysregulated state in the therapy, too. You may be in hyperarousal or maybe hypoarousal. You were probably not paying attention to your state and were unaware of it, but these dysregulated states influence your mind and body. That is not uncommon; that happens to all of us sometimes. What do you think about what I said?

The supervisor decided to use psychoeducation, explanation, and normalisation of the supervisee's states to strengthen the feeling of support and encourage the supervisee's reflection and emerging insight.

Supervisee: Yes, I want to bring more attention to my states, to my body within the therapy ... to see what I am feeling. If that's true, no wonder that I feel between the therapy sessions that she is too much.

Supervisor: Yes, I also think that the first step towards moving the therapy from its present stagnation and to reach a place where the client won't be too much for you is to observe your body state, be aware of it and regulate yourself and the client. If you are sensing a dysregulated state within yourself, probably the client is also in a dysregulated state. Go with the pace that you both can manage.

The supervisor explains and directs the supervisee to slow down the pace and make space for mindful awareness. Actually, what she proposed to the supervisee is the same as she did at the beginning of the supervision session when she was also annoyed by the supervisee's fast rhythm. Then she stopped the dysfunctional physiological synchronisation with her and regulated herself and the supervisee. The supervisor was modelling, in vivo, what the supervisee could do in the therapy.

Supervisee: *Yes, it makes more sense. Things are clearer now: about my sleep, the pain I was experiencing, feeling she is too much for me, the client not getting better.*
Supervisor: *What do you feel now in your body?*

The supervisor wants to integrate the supervisee's insight with her embodied awareness. She also models for the supervisee how to integrate cognitive and physiological dimensions in the therapy.

Supervisee: *I can breathe more easily, and I feel lighter. The pain is gone.*

With this regulated physiological state and new insights, the supervisee transforms her relational schema of being with her client. Based on that, she has a higher chance of entering the following therapy session in a renewed state of being, enabling her to stay present in the therapy and choose effective therapeutic interventions. This is what we want to accomplish in the process of supervision.

The vignette shows how the therapist was not mindfully aware of her inner states during the therapy sessions with her client. By being unaware, the therapist could not regulate either her own or her client's dysregulated states. The therapy was going in circles, the client's state was not improving, and the therapist developed physical symptoms (pain, sleeplessness) and resistance towards the client. In the presented session, the supervisor helps the supervisee regulate, come into contact with herself, and gain insight into the relational dynamic between her and the client. The supervisor accomplishes this by slowing the pace and encouraging mindful awareness of the supervisee's body. When the client and the therapist are in a hurry during the therapy session, they are too fast and lose contact with themselves. It is a paradox; the quicker they are, the more the therapy stagnates. By slowing down in supervision, we overcome the therapy stagnation. Decelerating in supervision is modelling the therapist on how to slow down and encourage regulation in the course of therapy. Supervision, in this way, aims to help the therapist and (through regulating the therapist) the client return to the window tolerance.

In the vignette, we can observe another relational dynamic between the client and the therapist Tanja. The client was unconsciously searching for care, and the therapist was giving "all of her" to the client. This corresponds with her history when Tanja was taking psychological care of her mother as a child. Based on her past personal relationships, the therapist has a dysfunctional relational schema "I should give everything to clients". According to that schema, she thinks that turning attention to herself and taking care of herself (by regulation) means "leaving" the client alone. The activation of this schema hinders the therapy process. By wanting to please the client, our therapist Tanja was losing contact with herself and was unaware of her merging and synchronising with the client's dysregulated physiology. Supervision helped her doubt the schema "I should give everything to clients", but since it was so connected with unresolved issues from the past, Tanja needed to work on that dysfunctional relational schema in her personal psychotherapy.

From both vignettes and other supervision cases from our practice, we have seen many times that therapists are not aware of their bodies and physiological states in their therapy work. They are unaware of their inner body/ physiological state when they merge with the client and are absorbed by them. Then they lose contact with themselves. Maintaining mindful body awareness is an essential tool that brings the therapist back into contact with themselves and into a balanced position in the relationship with their client.

The therapist's task is to regulate the client or help them to regulate themselves. For that task, a clear sense of boundary between the therapist and the client is needed. If we support the therapist in being mindfully aware of their inner states, they will also build functional boundaries between themselves and their clients.

Somebody has to discontinue dysregulated emotional and physiological circles. If the therapist does not do this, it is the supervisor's task to break this dysregulated pattern. They can accomplish this with the help of the supervision tasks of the Triple R model: Recognition, Regulation, and Reflection.

Chapter 10

Compassion-focused interventions in integrative supervision

In the song, High tide or low tide, Bob Marley narrates how he heard his mother crying and praying for her newborn child, who had come into this world. She asks God for protection and receives lovely words telling her that God will be the child's friend and be by his side no matter the circumstances – in high or low seas or in high or low tide.

Faith in something higher than us, who takes care of us, protects, guides, and loves us, is a powerful resource in our lives. As we can have a strong bond with the transpersonal source, we can also have a loving and kind relationship within ourselves. Whether we are up or down, in success or failure, in high tide or low tide, in any circumstance, we can have a powerful, stable, and accepting bond with ourselves. Anytime, anywhere, we have this possibility to be friends with ourselves, to be by our side. The song, in our opinion, represents the essence of compassion and self-compassion processes.

An analysis of the song's words (child, born, cry, a plea for protection) also indicates who awakens God's love and compassion: The innocent, vulnerable, and humble. We can understand these words in this way: To arouse compassion in others or invoke self-compassion, we first need to get in touch with vulnerability. In supervision, when we want the supervisee to regain their compassion towards the client, we lead them into seeing their client as innocent, vulnerable, or as a child. When we promote the supervisee's self-compassion, we also help them to see their vulnerability.

Compassion involves the intention that a person in pain is relieved from their suffering. In a compassionate state, we are open to others' painful experiences, willing for their suffering to touch us. The compassionate state is connected to warmth, wishing others well, tolerance, and wisdom (Germer, 2012). Compassion naturally arises when we can look at other people or ourselves through the eyes of the observing self; from a wider perspective uncoloured by our personal schemas. All three mindful processes are necessary for compassion: Present moment awareness, acceptance, and decentred perspective.

Neff (2003a, 2011) defines three main components of self-compassion: Self-kindness, common humanity, and mindfulness. Self-compassion brings kindness towards ourselves when experiencing pain and helps us to understand that

DOI: 10.4324/9781003194118-13

our imperfections, pain, and suffering are part of our common human experience. Psychotherapists are often very critical and judgmental towards themselves and sometimes have difficulty relating to themselves with kindness and love (M. Žvelc, 2017). While they may be, on the one hand, entirely dedicated to their clients, they often fail to treat themselves with the same level of respect and dignity. Enhancing self-compassion helps psychotherapists to develop a nurturing and loving inner relationship, a cornerstone of mental health and prevention against burnout. The loving inner relationship is beneficial in psychotherapy, as it brings a compassionate presence to the psychotherapy relationship. Such presence helps the psychotherapist to self-regulate, contain painful emotions and relate with care to their clients.

Mindfulness and self-compassion are interwoven processes (Germer & Neff, 2013). They represent the way we relate to ourselves and our experiences. Mindfulness encompasses compassion and compassion mindfulness. But in a narrower sense, we can say that mindfulness relates to accepting awareness of our experience, while self-compassion relates to the acceptance of the experiencer. People often do not just avoid or refuse their experiences; they judge themselves for having those experiences.

This chapter presents how to promote compassion and self-compassion within supervision sessions. Situations occurring during psychotherapy are emotionally demanding and often stressful for psychotherapists. Therapists are empathic to their clients, which is desirable, but feeling the emotions of others in pain increases the experience of negative affect and can lead to empathic distress (Klimecki et al., 2013). However, empathy combined with mindfulness and compassion increases positive affect, may strengthen resilience and emotional regulation strategies, and keep therapists from empathic distress (Klimecki & Singer, 2012; Leonard et al., 2018). Research also shows self-compassion as a significant protective factor against burnout among healthcare professionals (Atkinson et al., 2017; Eriksson et al., 2018; Kastelic et al., 2022; Kotera et al., 2021; Richardson et al., 2020). Self-compassion correlates positively with emotional regulation (Barlow et al., 2017; Bates et al., 2021; Diedrich et al., 2016; Finlay-Jones, 2017; Inwood & Ferrari, 2018; Scoglio et al., 2015; Vettese et al., 2011) and negatively with shame and self-criticism (Sedighimornani et al., 2019). Safran et al. (2008) emphasise that supervisees need to have the capacity of self-acceptance so that they can explore themselves and their experiences, from their weaknesses to their strengths. Based on these findings and our own clinical practice, we emphasise the importance of promoting compassion and self-compassion in supervision.

Supervisor's compassion towards supervisees and their clients

The supervisor's compassionate attitude, which shows openness, warmth, and empathy towards supervisees and their clients (M. Žvelc, 2015, 2017) and humility (Watkins et al., 2019), is a crucial facilitative factor in supervision.

The supervisor's compassion provides a safe supervisory environment and prevents harm in a supervisory relationship (McCrea & Bulanda, 2008). Supervisees internalise the compassionate attitude of their supervisors and convey it to their clients. Internalising a compassionate attitude helps supervisees develop a compassionate internal supervisor (Coaston, 2019).

Supervisor's lack of compassion

Sometimes, the supervisor may lack a compassionate attitude toward the supervisee or their clients (M. Žvelc, 2017). In this case, the supervisor's mindful awareness is needed to recognise this. We suggest the supervisor observes their feelings mindfully and tries to understand their impatience. There is a reason why the supervisor feels a lack of compassion. As a young psychotherapist, I (Maša) remember that once in a supervision session, I found my supervisor very critical of one of my clients. At that time, I had quite a strong motherhood transference toward this client, and the supervisor's condemnatory and disapproving attitude toward my client bothered me. I told him that I found him very critical and condemning of my client. At this point, our supervisory alliance was at stake. The supervisor thought about what I had said and admitted I was right, that he did feel irritation towards my client, and he explained why. The client was in psychotherapy education, and my supervisor was upset with some of her immature behaviour, which did not seem appropriate for a future psychotherapist. He also revealed that he had doubts about the institute that was responsible for her education. For me, his disclosure was vital; our alliance not only repaired but even grew stronger. I felt I could trust him, continue discussing therapy with the client, and keep bringing this case to supervision. It was significant that dysregulated, unspoken supervisor's affect, which lacked compassion for my client, was brought to awareness and communicated between him and me as a supervisee.

This anecdote also shows how supervisees are aware of the supervisor's attitude toward their clients. The supervisor being disrespectful and lacking compassion for the clients can result in the supervisee not disclosing that particular therapy case or even dropping out of supervision (M. Žvelc, 2017; M. Žvelc & Žvelc, 2021).

Supervisee's compassion toward their clients

A psychotherapist's willingness to be touched by their client's suffering and being able to feel and convey compassion for the client's suffering is essential for effective psychotherapy. In a compassionate response, the therapist attunes to the client beyond empathy (Erskine, 2020), decentres themselves from feeling the same as the client, and offers a reciprocal response (Erskine, 2020; Uršič & Žvelc, 2017). With the therapist's attitude of compassion, the client feels understood, supported, and safe. Sometimes it is challenging for the therapist to find compassion for their client. In supervision, we help the therapist recognise their lack of compassion, understand its causes, normalise it, and, if appropriate, help regain their compassion.

Supervisee's lack of compassion

Therapists generally have a high capacity for being compassionate to their clients. But there are some situations when they find this difficult. Different factors contribute to this. It may happen when the client commits actions in their life that the therapist resents and cannot accept the client as a person. For instance, this happens if the client admits that they have sexually abused their child, hit their partner or done other such acts. Sometimes client's behaviour may not be morally or ethically objectionable but nevertheless irritates the therapist. For example, some supervisees have difficulties accepting clients who always want to be at the centre of attention, clients who praise themselves a lot, clients who are passive and distant, clients in a particular religion or with a particular political or sociocultural opinion which contradicts the therapist's views. The therapist can also have difficulties with acceptance and compassion when clients exhibit an attitude and behaviour in the therapy session which is hurtful, such as aggressiveness and humiliating the psychotherapist. The inability to feel acceptance and compassion towards their client is a part of the therapist's countertransference. It depends on the interaction of the client's behaviour and the therapist's relational schemas triggered by the client's acts. In supervision, we help the supervisee explore factors contributing to a lack of compassion toward the client. In some cases, especially at the outset of psychotherapy, when the formal psychotherapy contract has not yet been made, we may discuss whether the therapist should take the person in psychotherapy. In other cases, we help the therapist to understand their reaction and (re)gain compassion for the client.

When a psychotherapist feels attacked, humiliated, ignored, or in other ways suffers in their relationship with the client, their capacity for mindful awareness and compassion narrows. The therapist, in such cases, activates their survival mechanisms. Wounded, they protect themselves. Here the role of supervision is vital. Supervision helps therapists recognise the relational enactment they are caught in and helps them to step out of it (Frawley-O'Dea & Sarnat, 2001). Mindful awareness in supervision allows therapists to regain contact with themselves and their clients and feel compassionate when needed. We want to stress that we do not promote feelings of compassion all the time or at any cost. It is normal and inevitable that the therapist will have a range of emotions in relation to the client. But what is essential is that the psychotherapist stays grounded and present, within the window of tolerance, while with the client. And that they can feel compassion when the client reveals their vulnerability and pain.

Sometimes the therapist lacks compassion for most of their clients. The therapist may feel clients are a burden; they may not be interested in their clients' stories and struggles. Clients' suffering becomes too much for them, or they become so distant that the clients' pain does not touch them. Such cases may show that the therapist is tired and worn out and that they are probably experiencing empathic distress or burnout. In this case, the therapist needs more self-care. We write about different aspects of self-care in Chapter 12.

Helping the supervisee to regain compassion toward their client

The supervisor can help the supervisee to regain compassion toward their clients in different ways: 1) By raising the supervisee's mindful awareness of the client's suffering, and 2) By raising the supervisee's mindful awareness of their own suffering triggered by the psychotherapy work.

Compassion is often invoked by inviting the supervisee to contact their observing self and mindfully observing the client or themselves from the position of a loving witness.

Raising the supervisee's mindful awareness of the client's suffering

The supervisor can focus the supervisee's attention on painful events in their client's current life, their suffering because of the symptoms, or their painful history. They can also help the supervisee reframe the client's "mistakes" using the common humanity concept.

When the supervisor focuses the supervisee on the client's suffering, they can help the supervisee realise that behind the client's irritable behaviour, there is a wound, a need for protection, and a need for attachment. The client's behaviour has a reason behind it and a story to tell.

The supervisor may assist the supervisee in imagining the client as a child, seeing their wounds and suffering, seeing their vulnerable body postures, and realising which coping mechanism they had to create to survive. With this, we elicit compassion. Then the supervisee can see the client's irritable behaviour not as acts that diminish them but as the old ways of protection. Furthermore, they may realise that something in the therapy made the client feel unsafe, so they had to activate their protective mechanisms in the therapeutic relationship.

To lead the supervisee to see the client as an innocent or a vulnerable child, we can use the following exercise that utilises active imagination:

"Imagine standing in front of a closed door which leads to a room. In the room, there is a little girl/boy_____ (name of the client). Slowly open the door. Look around; notice what do you see or hear? (We give time for the supervisee to do this. Let the supervisee tell you answers out loud.) *Do you see_____ (name of the client) as a child? How does she/he look?* (Let the supervisee

describe the child in detail). *What posture does she/he have?* (Seeing a child in a vulnerable posture universally awakes compassion) *What is she/he doing? What do you experience now when looking at her/him?"*

Often it is enough to lead the supervisee to this point. Seeing the client as a child, often lonely or scared, in a vulnerable body posture is likely to evoke compassion in the therapist. Seeing a child happy, playing, jumping or smiling may enable a supervisee to associate with the child's innocence, which may also stir a gentle and compassionate response in the supervisee. As a supervisor, we may want to continue the exercise and lead the supervisee to explore the relationship with the imagined child and lead to an interaction with them:

"Did she/he notice you? (If yes), how did she/he react? Would you like to take a step closer? Would you like to tell something to her/him or make body contact? What is happening now? What does the girl/boy do?"

We lead the supervisee slowly, letting them develop their imagination by themselves. We are careful not to intrude on the supervisee or the imagined child. From this exploration, the dynamic between the psychotherapist and the client may become more evident; the therapist understands the client's needs and pain more profoundly, and sometimes they touchingly connect in their imagination.

After this exercise, we may ask the supervisee to imagine the next therapy session with that client and what they are experiencing now. Usually, after this experience, they feel their defensive shield is gone; they soften, feeling more warm, open, and compassionate towards the client and ready for the session.

We learned similar exercises at the International Integrative Psychotherapy Association (IIPA) conference at one of the workshops (Senior & Shotter, 2007). I (Maša) volunteered to be supervised by one of the workshop leaders. I selected a client Patricia, with whom I felt uncomfortable. The client was highly motivated for psychotherapy but also very controlling. I experienced her as if she watched my every move, which for me was quite repulsive. My body, in her presence, stiffened. From previous supervision, I realised that she was behaving as her parents did in relation to her. They were very controlling and strict; she was afraid of making almost any move, was anxious, and later developed obsessions and compulsions. The control of the client made me feel uncomfortable. Although I understood why, this was not enough to significantly change my body reactions and the way of being with the client. The workshop leader led me through a similar process to the exercise described above. I saw my client, approximately five years old, alone in a nicely furnished room with big windows shaded by heavy curtains, preventing the sunlight from entering. I was surprised by how quickly I felt sadness in my body. I thought to myself – aha, Patricia might be carrying a lot of sorrow. Previously, I was not aware of that; we were more directed toward exploring her fear and anger.

As I saw it in my imagination, the room symbolised the environment in which she lived and her inner world: Everything proper, but empty, alone, with obstacles to light and joy. I sensed the pain, which subsequently roused my warmth and compassion. In the following therapy session, I was different. I waited for her with warmth and openness; my body was soft and relaxed. If not consciously, she might have noticed my change through physiological synchrony. In the session, she managed to break out of the ties that bound her; she cried for the first time in therapy. Her crying was deep and touching.

That was probably the first time I profoundly realised how essential the therapist's way of being with the client is. We have a powerful tool in supervision in transforming the therapist's protective mechanisms into awareness and compassion.

Raising the supervisee's mindful awareness of their own suffering, triggered by the psychotherapy work

In supervision, the supervisee may also need to explore their personal wounds triggered by the client's story or behaviour. As psychotherapists, we are always influenced by our clients, whether or not we are aware of it. Usually, the client's characteristic, which the therapist cannot accept, is connected to a lack of self-acceptance by the therapist in some areas. In this case, we lead the supervisee from impatience towards the client to mindful awareness and reflection of their own wounds. These wounds can be from the present time, adulthood, or past, childhood or adolescence. When being mindful of their pain, the supervisee usually discovers that what they cannot tolerate within the client, they do not tolerate within themselves and was probably not tolerated by significant others when they were a child. When the supervisees regain compassion towards themselves in some specific area, compassion towards the client usually arises spontaneously. This kind of supervision work is strongly associated with work on countertransference.

Vignette: "I can't stand the client's demands for attention"

The supervisee, Tanya, was often irritated by some features of one of her clients. In various situations in her life, the client wanted to have a lot of attention and be in the centre and was very offended when she wasn't. After one psychotherapy session, Tanya was particularly upset by her client's behaviour. To Tanya, the client's conduct was childish and irresponsible. For Tanya, the client acted like a five-year girl; she "forced" others to give her a lot of attention. Tanya's countertransference reaction was strong; she was angry at the client, judging her. At that moment in this supervision session, she was merged with her experience, lacking optimal distance to her inner world.

I (Maša), as supervisor, wanted to regulate her by slowing down the rhythm and raising mindful bodily awareness. I asked her what she was experiencing. She felt a faster heartbeat, pressure in her chest, and irritation in her arms and legs. She exhaled deeply and slowed down a little. Then I invited her to participate in an exercise, which included exploring her being a child. She agreed. I asked her to close her eyes, be aware of her body sensations here and now, and let her mind take her to the flat where she lived when she was five. At a slow pace, step by step, I started to enquire what she was seeing, who was in the apartment, and what was happening.

Through her body sensations, I trusted that her mind would bridge from present to past and take her to a meaningful scene in childhood. She first saw her mother tired after work and busy in the kitchen. Then she turned her gaze to her brother. He is preparing to go out to play with friends from the neighbourhood. She is looking at him. She would like to go with him; she would like him to take her with him. She is quiet; she does not tell him this. She knows he wouldn't want her to go with him even if she asked him to. As a supervisor, I wished her to find her voice, to find her words, to find and accept her needs. I said to her: "*What would you like to tell him? What would your body like to do?*" She became aware of her need and was able to verbalise it strongly: "*I would like to go out with you. I want to play with you and your friends*". And then she demanded: "*Take me with me!*"

Supervisor: *What do you feel now?*
Supervisee Tanya: *A feeling of power in my hands.*

Here we finished the exercise; the personal experience so far was enough for the supervision aims, and we started to reflect on it.

The supervisee, Tanya, got in touch with her previous "not allowed" need to be seen and to be taken into account; to be significant to the others close to her, and to demand something from them. She realised that she suppressed that need. Now she felt she had the right to wish others would pay attention to her and to express her need or wish. She felt softness and kindness towards the little girl.

Then we connected her experience and insights with her countertransference response to her client. We discussed how she might envy the client, who lets herself demand attention. She realised that the two of them represented two sides of the same coin: One craving and demanding, the other too restricted. Within both, there was probably the pain of neglect.

Accepting her need for attention as a normal relational need, the psychotherapist Tanya could also soften and open in the relationship with her client; she could be more tolerant towards the client's hunger for attention, which she previously experienced just as childish and selfish neediness. She felt compassion towards the client and knew in what direction to continue the psychotherapy: To help the client find her original pain and help her to value the need for attention, but ask for it in a socially acceptable way and not in a way which drives others away.

Not forcing compassion

When we notice impatience and the lack of compassion in the supervisee, we do not try to impose compassion at any cost. Compassion is genuine if it emerges naturally from within the person. We, as supervisors, may only encourage this inner source to flow.

As is shown in the above vignette, it can be beneficial if a supervisor encourages self-compassion in the supervisee towards the suffering they experience with the clients. With this process, their protective mechanisms soften, and they can become compassionate towards themselves and their clients. Sometimes, the psychotherapy with the clients triggers unprocessed trauma, and the flow of compassion in the supervisee may become stuck. Then we discuss with the supervisee about addressing these issues in their personal psychotherapy.

Compassionate confrontation

Sometimes people think that being compassionate means complying and approving. In compassion for others, we do not need to agree with them. In supervision, there are situations when the supervisor disagrees with the supervisee, does not see the supervisee's interventions as effective, or evaluates some supervisee's decisions as wrong or unethical. The supervisor's role is to give clear feedback to the supervisee, and sometimes, this feedback is challenging.

Supervision is a situation where the supervisee exposes their work, including shortcomings, gaps, fears, and doubts. In this way, the supervisee can learn and develop. At the same time, this exposure can lead to feelings of vulnerability and shame (Alonso & Rutan, 1988; Talbot, 1995).

The supervision function is also about monitoring the quality of the supervisee's work and serves as a gatekeeper to the profession (Bernard & Goodyear, 2013), which further heightens the supervisee's anxiety and feeling vulnerable. It is important that, as supervisors, we are aware of this, that we are attuned to our supervisees' vulnerability and remain respectful when giving supervisees challenging feedback or setting them boundaries.

When providing challenging feedback, we advise supervisors to do this mindfully and with compassion. When the supervisor does not agree with the supervisee or is not satisfied with some of the supervisee's actions, we advise them to use the mindful pause to become aware of their feelings. If they notice their physiology is dysregulated, or they are agitated, angry, and outside the window of tolerance, they may want to ground themselves and use slower breathing before giving feedback to the supervisee. If they have difficulties regulating, it may be better for the supervisor to postpone the feedback and talk to their own supervisor first to process their elevated feelings. In Chapter 5, when presenting the hindering moments in supervision, we can see that some supervisors are too quick and reckless in their response and humiliate their supervisees (M. Žvelc, 2017).

If the supervisor is grounded and within the window of tolerance, they can attune to the supervisee's feelings and needs. They can give the supervisee challenging feedback from that present and compassionate state. The essential elements of this kind of feedback are: Giving the supervisee concrete feedback with respect to the supervisee as a person and as a professional.

Below are two examples of giving challenging feedback from our supervision practice: Initial confrontative feedback from an emotionally dysregulated and not compassionate state and confrontative feedback from the state of presence, respect, and compassion.

Vignette: Supervisor's feedback from a non-compassionate state: "I do not like your intervention"

The supervisee, Barbara, shared with her supervisor that she had confronted her client regarding his passivity in his life. The supervisor disagreed with this intervention. She felt agitated and frustrated with this way of pushing the client; it was not her working style. She told the supervisee that she did not see this kind of intervention as helpful and wondered how the client felt. She tried to be calm and respectful. But the supervisee felt the supervisor's irritation and started to defend herself. After a few minutes, they both became angrier, and the conversation was going in circles. At that moment, there was a clear rupture in the alliance. The supervisor realised that they both needed to take a step back. She initiated a mindful pause and asked the supervisee, with genuine interest, what she was feeling. The supervisee shared that she was angry. The supervisor admitted that she was angry, too. While pausing and sharing, their physiology and emotions slowed down, and they started using the social engagement system (Porges, 2017). They metacommunicated how those past few minutes were for them and regained their alliance. After that, they explored what may be the meaning of their relational impasse. With the help of mindful awareness and compassion towards each other, they could sincerely understand one another, the repair was done, and they could continue the supervision within the window of tolerance, where integration of new learning is possible.

Vignette: The supervisor's confrontation with compassion: "I wonder, how come you used this intervention?"

The supervisee, Susan, complains that her client, whenever she asks what he is feeling, always answers with words like "I don't know, nothing". While listening to the tape of the psychotherapy session with him, the supervisor notices that Susan has a stern, teacher-like voice while talking to her client. When asking the client what he is feeling now, her voice becomes cold. The supervisor is surprised because she knows Susan as a warm person with a good capacity for attunement. She hypothesises that Susan's restrained attitude has a meaning and probably serves as a protective function. The supervisor feels warmth and compassion toward Susan. She gives her feedback: "*I know you can be warm to your clients. In this tape, your voice is different from usual, more strict and cold. I think* (pause) *if you ask the client what he feels with this kind of voice, no wonder he cannot come into touch with his feelings. How do you see what I have just told you?*" Susan agrees that her voice is indeed cold. In the subsequent discussion, she realises that she is afraid that if her client does come into touch with his feelings, they might be powerful, and she might not know what to do then. She realises that, in some way, she was cold and strict to protect him from getting into contact with his inner experience and that she was also protecting herself.

From the vignette, we can see that the supervisor provided the feedback in a way which offered clear information and, at the same time, respect and safety. The feedback did not threaten the supervisee. The supervisee felt safe and open to exploring her experience and the meaning of her behaviour. That was crucial in this supervision session.

Self-compassion-focused interventions in supervision

In this chapter, we have so far discussed promoting the supervisor's compassion towards the supervisee and the client, and the supervisee's compassion towards the client. We have seen how the supervisee's compassion towards themselves could encourage compassion for clients. In this last part of the chapter and the next chapter, we exclusively focus on promoting the supervisee's self-compassion in supervision. Promoting self-compassion in supervisees can lessen their self-criticism and other distress connected to their work and improve their work as therapists (Coaston, 2019).

We, as professional helpers, may not be aware of just how stressful and challenging it can be to work with people with problems and witness a lot of suffering. We may not recognise how we come to absorb the client's pain and stress like a sponge and hold it in our psyche and body. Self-compassion helps us to overcome the harm this causes us and awakes our caring and loving attention towards ourselves as professionals, recognising our struggles, discomfort, and suffering, and giving ourselves gentle care and support. We are not alone; we all have struggles and difficulties at work, self-criticism, feelings of powerlessness or hopelessness, and other strong emotions. Many of us experience our clients' aggressiveness, contempt, ignorance, suicide or suicidal attempts. All these situations often leave us suffering.

If we have (enough) compassion toward ourselves, we can promote compassion for others without exhausting ourselves. Newsome et al. (2012) proposed that effectiveness as a helper might be linked to the ability to be self-compassionate.

There are various ways to promote self-compassion (Desmond, 2016; Germer & Neff, 2013; P. Gilbert, 2010; Neff, 2011; G. Žvelc & Žvelc, 2021), and some of them we have adapted to our supervision work.

In MCIS, we promote self-compassion in three main ways:

1 Enhancing self-compassion with relational methods within the attuned supervisory relationship.
2 The use of self-compassion exercises.
3 Self-compassionate processing.

Enhancing self-compassion with relational methods within the attuned supervisory relationship

In MCIS, we promote the supervisee's self-compassion during the supervision session within an attuned supervisory relationship. We believe self-compassion is an inner state existing and reachable to all of us. A compassionate supervisor can help the supervisee to find and bring this internal resource to the surface.

For enhancing self-compassion, we use the keyhole model of relational mindfulness and compassion (see Chapter 2, Figure 2.3). We integrated the original Erskine keyhole model (Erskine, 2015; Erskine & Trautmann, 1997) with mindfulness and compassion processes (G. Žvelc & Žvelc, 2021) and adapted it for use in supervision. The keyhole model includes interventions that enhance mindfulness and compassion within an attuned psychotherapy relationship. In Chapter 7, we describe how the model is used to promote mindfulness processes: Present moment awareness, acceptance, and decentred perspective. These processes are essential for helping the supervisee become aware of and accept their suffering. Interventions of *inquiry* and *acknowledgement* of the supervisee's experience raise awareness of suffering, while the intervention of *validation* promotes its acceptance. For self-compassion, *normalisation* is crucial, being the intervention that encourages the experience of common humanity. The supervisor's presence and attunement help these methods to be used at the right time and in a way that promotes safety and facilitates the supervision process. In addition to these methods, the supervisor leads the supervisee to relate from the observing self and find the loving witness decentred position.

In MCIS, we first want to enhance the supervisees' mindful awareness of their suffering with phenomenological inquiry, acknowledgement, and validation of their experience. Then we evoke self-compassion by inviting the supervisee to mindfully observe themselves from the position of a loving witness and bring kindness towards themselves. The therapist may say: *"Just look at yourself in the session when you were feeling shame"*. And then we encourage the supervisee to look at themselves with loving eyes: *"Look at yourself with loving eyes, as you would be looking at a person, whom you deeply care about"*. Seeing themselves in pain from the position of a loving witness naturally evokes self-compassion. The supervisor may then invite the supervisee to self-compassionate dialogue with themselves: *"What would you like to say to yourself? What words of compassion would you like to convey to yourself?"*

Apart from developing kindness towards self or others, common humanity is another quality essential to self-compassion (Neff, 2003a, 2011). The important aspect of conveying common humanity is through the supervisory relationship itself. In the keyhole model of relational mindfulness and compassion, the primary way to convey common humanity is through the intervention of normalisation. For the effectiveness of this intervention, it is important that the supervisee is already mindfully aware of their pain, which is promoted by interventions of phenomenological inquiry, acknowledgement, and validation. While phenomenological inquiry and acknowledgement promote present-moment awareness, and validation enhances acceptance, the intervention of normalisation goes one step further. Normalisation conveys to the supervisee that their experience is a normal and not pathological reaction. Normalisation de-pathologises the person's definition of their internal experiences or coping mechanisms (Erskine, 2015). This intervention is related to the fundamental principle of mindfulness- and compassion-oriented integrative psychotherapy that people experience *ordinary unhappiness*, which means that they are not perfect, experience pain, and sometimes make unwise decisions (M. Žvelc & Žvelc, 2021).

In the following example, we see how the supervisor promotes the supervisee's self-compassion by normalisation of the supervisee's experience.

Supervisee:	*I feel so much shame regarding the last session with Rebecca. I started to cry in the middle of the session. She talked about the loss of her mother, and I could not help myself. Tears just came, and I just could not stop them.*
Supervisor:	*How do you feel now?*
Supervisee (looks away from the therapist):	*I feel shame and that you will think of me that I am a bad therapist who cannot control herself.*
Supervisor (with a warm voice):	*The tears were a natural response to the pain your client was experiencing. They are significant and valuable.*

The supervisor conveys the normalisation of tears as a common human experience when we see a person suffering. As the supervisee experiences shame that involves self-criticism, normalisation may provide an antidote in the form of self-compassion. The supervisor also invites acceptance of her tears with the intervention of validation, saying they are significant and valuable.

Supervisee: *I feel touched by your words. I was criticising myself heavily before, and now I feel relief … . (pause) I still wonder if this was helpful to my client.*

The supervisee seems more compassionate to herself and now looks at the session from a professional perspective.

Supervisor: *How did your client respond?*
Supervisee: *She said that she is touched that someone is impacted by her loss.*
Supervisor: *Become aware of her words. What do you feel inside when you hear that? Just take a moment and observe your experience. (mindful pause) What comes up?*
Supervisee: *Relief and feeling calm. And the thought that I am not the worst therapist! (smiles) I feel more accepting towards myself as a person and as a professional.*

It seems that the supervisee's emotional reaction may actually have been helpful for the client. What the supervisee considered a big mistake was helpful for the client, who could see that someone was impacted by their suffering. The need to have an impact is a significant relational need (Erskine, 2015). The supervisor invited the supervisee to be mindful of the client's words, which enhanced the supervisee's self-acceptance.

Normalisation of the supervisee's experience may also be focused on the coping strategies of the supervisee. Supervisees often blame themselves for their coping strategies used in the psychotherapy session. In the case of a supervisee who dissociated during the session because their client was describing sexual abuse in detail, the supervisor said: "*I imagine that this was really painful, so going away emotionally helped you to navigate the session till the end*".

In conveying normalisation, it is important that the supervisor is present and compassionate, which is expressed in a kind tone of voice and with soft facial expressions.

Self-compassion exercises

In addition to these relational interventions that are part of the keyhole model of relational mindfulness and compassion, self-compassion can also be enhanced by self-compassion exercises. The supervisor can propose that supervisees do self-compassionate exercises at home or at the beginning of supervision sessions. We often integrate some of these exercises into the supervision work during the supervision session, especially as a part of self-compassion processing, when we want to encourage the supervisee's self-compassion. It is also beneficial when supervisees attend structured self-compassion programmes (Bell et al., 2017; Germer & Neff, 2013; Newsome et al., 2012).

Below we introduce four self-compassion exercises that we have found to be very effective and use most often in our daily lives, therapy, training, and supervision. We suggest trying them first by yourselves before introducing them to supervisees. They may be done at the beginning of the supervision/psychotherapy session or at any moment of suffering during the supervision/psychotherapy session. The exercises are also a valuable tool for emotional and physiological regulation and can be used when the supervisor wants to regulate themselves or the supervisee. While leading the exercise, the supervisor's voice is soft and gentle, and the pace of speaking is slow.

Loving hand

"Put your hand on your chest in a kind and loving way. Feel the touch of your hand; feel the warmth of your hand on your chest. Be aware of the gentle, loving, accepting touch. Feel the touch of your hand on your heart, the touch of love, compassion, and forgiveness".[1]

The Loving hand exercise includes a self-soothing touch and promotes a compassionate interaction with the body. The gentle and soothing touch is at the root of self-compassion and encourages the bottom-up process of self-compassion. It conveys support and feelings of safety. A soothing touch raises oxytocin levels, reduces cortisol response to stress and other stress responses and increases positive attitudes and bonding (Arch et al., 2014; Dreisoerner et al., 2021; Uvnäs-Moberg et al., 2014). A similar exercise is also presented in other publications (Germer, 2012; van der Brink & Koster, 2015).

Supporting breath

"Direct your attention to your breathing. The in-breath ... the out-breath ... . Be aware, that every single breath is supporting you, is here with you ... cares for you ... supplying the oxygen to your body, to the cells ... giving you the energy, the strength you need ... and taking away waste substances ... Be aware of your breath; the supporting and caring nature of your breath ... being with you throughout your life".[2]

Breathing is a vital function that is under our voluntary control, and by influencing breathing, we can also impact our physiology, emotions, and cognition (Ley, 1994). In the exercise, we remind a person that they are taken care of and supported by their breathing, which accompanies them all the time. The exercise raises the level of feeling safe, relaxes the muscles connected to breathing, and optimises the person's breathing. The supporting breath exercise is inspired by part of Jon Kabat-Zinn's body scan meditation.

Loving-kindness body scan

> "Sitting in a comfortable position, feeling your body, your back, your buttocks and your legs pressing on the chair or the floor; feeling their weight, sensing their gravity. Feeling how you are supported, held by the chair, by the floor. Feeling the Earth is holding you and supporting you.
> Breathing; long in-breath, prolonged out-breath.
> Being aware of your body. Scanning your body from your toes to your head.
> Noticing any tension, breathe into that part of your body with love and kindness, and release the strain with the out-breath. Repeat that with every region of the body where it's not comfortable; breathing in that part, caressing it with loving and kindness".

The Loving-kindness body scan exercise combines mindful body awareness with loving and compassionate breath. Awareness of gravity helps a person to ground themselves. The sense that something (the object, the Earth) is holding them provides a feeling of safety, that they can lean on and release some of their control. Awareness of the body brings a person into deep internal contact, and by compassionate breath, they build a loving bond with their body and themselves as a whole. The exercise is inspired by Tara Brach (Brach, 2020), and the body scan meditation and lake meditation from Jon Kabat-Zinn.

Self-compassion phrase

> "When you are in distress and suffering in any way, it may help you to gently, lovingly say these words to yourself:
> _____ (saying your name), this is a moment of suffering,
> _____ (saying your name), be kind to yourself.
> You can support this self-compassion phrase by lovingly putting your hand on your chest".

This exercise is an adaptation of the exercise presented by Neff (2011, p. 119). It combines part of her self-compassion phrase exercise with the loving hand exercise. The self-compassion phrase exercise includes a self-compassionate internal dialogue. It promotes mindful awareness of a person's suffering and a compassionate phrase, which conveys kindness and love to the person. The use of the loving hand exercise additionally grounds self-compassion in the body and promotes self-regulation.

After implementing the exercise, the supervisor asks the supervisee: "*What are you experiencing right now?*" or "*How was that exercise for you?*"

Supervisees can also write a self-compassionate letter to themselves from the view of a supportive and wise imagined supervisor (Coaston, 2019). In this way, they develop an internal compassionate dialogue with themselves and develop a compassionate internal supervisor (Bell et al., 2017; Coaston, 2019).

We have described two ways of promoting self-compassion in supervision. The first relates to enhancing self-compassion with relational methods within the supervisory relationship, and the second uses self-compassion exercises. In the next chapter, we describe a third way of promoting self-compassion in MCIS, a method of self-compassion processing. Self-compassion processing is a method for processing the supervisee's painful and dysregulated countertransference with the help of self-compassion.

Notes

1   Reprinted from *Integrative psychotherapy: A mindfulness- and compassion-oriented approach* (p. 148), by G. Žvelc & M. Žvelc, 2021, Routledge. Copyright 2021 by G. Žvelc & M. Žvelc. Reprinted with permission of the authors and the publisher (Taylor & Francis Ltd, www.tandfonline.com).

2   Reprinted from *Integrative psychotherapy: A mindfulness- and compassion-oriented approach* (p. 148), by G. Žvelc & M. Žvelc, 2021, Routledge. Copyright 2021 by G. Žvelc & M. Žvelc. Reprinted with permission of the authors and the publisher (Taylor & Francis Ltd, www.tandfonline.com).

Chapter 11

Self-compassion processing in supervision

In this chapter, we present the self-compassion processing supervision method and show how we use self-compassion to transform painful countertransference experiences. Self-compassion processing, originally used in mindfulness- and compassion-oriented integrative psychotherapy, aims to help a person process unresolved and painful issues and create a safe and loving bond within themselves (G. Žvelc & Žvelc, 2021). From this, we have designed a self-compassion processing method for supervision purposes.

In self-compassion processing, we are attentive to those stressful and challenging events which therapists may experience with their clients. Our aim is to revive the therapist's self-compassion so that they can face and transform their suffering with the help of this essential resource. We wish them to become aware of their pain and bring a kind and loving attitude to themselves. In this way, their painful countertransference is processed, and they can continue the psychotherapy process with their client in a new and present way.

The transformative power of self-compassion

Self-compassion processing starts with recognising certain markers. These markers include various signs that are indicative of the supervisee's painful and unprocessed countertransference experience: Self-criticism, shame, feelings of hurt, despair, uselessness, powerlessness, tiredness, meaningless, emptiness, and exhaustion. Markers also include signs of the supervisee's anxiety, urge to work hard, excessive worrying, and other painful experiences connected to their psychotherapy work. In the self-compassion processing method, the supervisor leads the supervisee into recognising their suffering, connected to their psychotherapy work, and helps them relate to themselves with care and self-compassion. In this way, the supervisee becomes a loving witness to their painful experiences and recreates a supporting and loving bond with themselves. Self-compassion processing enables emotional and physiological regulation of the supervisee's countertransference experience,

DOI: 10.4324/9781003194118-14

returning them to the window of tolerance where they can stay present, think flexibly, act optimally, and reconnect with their clients.

Connecting the supervisee's state of painful and unprocessed counter-transference experience with a self-compassionate state transforms how the supervisee feels and thinks about themselves, the client, and the initial problem brought to supervision. Compassion leads to transformation and integration of the mind (Desmond, 2016; P. Gilbert, 2010; G. Žvelc & Žvelc, 2021). We suggest that connecting the painful and disturbing counter-transference states with resourceful, mindful, and self-compassionate states leads to memory reconsolidation (Ecker et al., 2012; Ecker & Vaz, 2019). Self-compassion processing, in this way, transforms the supervisee's relational schemas of being with the client. It changes the supervisee's way of being at the supervision session and consequently in the subsequent psychotherapy sessions.

Phases of self-compassion processing in supervision

In self-compassion processing, there are three fundamental phases:

1 Leading the supervisee to mindful awareness of their painful experience.
2 Promoting the supervisee's self-compassion.

   2.1 Leading the supervisee to look at themselves with loving eyes from a bird's eye perspective.
   2.2 Promoting the supervisee's self-compassionate touch.
   2.3 Encouraging the supervisee's self-compassionate internal dialogue.

3 Integration

   3.1 Connecting the supervisee's new self-compassionate state to the supervision problem
   3.2 Reflection on the supervision process.

The first two phases are drawn from the basic principles for awakening self-compassion both in a person in general (Brach, 2012; Neff, 2011; R. D. Siegel & Germer, 2012) and also in psychotherapy (Desmond, 2016; Germer, 2012; P. Gilbert, 2010; G. Žvelc & Žvelc, 2021). We have adjusted them for supervision and added the third phase, integration. Integration is accomplished by connecting the supervisee's new self-compassionate state with the initial supervision problem and reflecting on the whole supervision process.

These phases are a guidance tool for the supervisor. Sometimes the phases and sub-phases are interwoven. The supervisor uses them flexibly and may also skip some of the subphases.

In the following pages, we first describe the phases of self-compassion processing and then illustrate them through two vignettes.

Phase 1: Leading the supervisee to mindful awareness of their painful experience

In this phase, the supervisor leads the supervisee to recognise and become mindfully aware of the specific moment of their suffering connected to their psychotherapy work. We lead supervisees to come into contact with the pain stemming from their work in a way that "they are not overwhelmed by it and not avoiding it, but are the loving witness to it" (G. Žvelc & Žvelc, 2021, p. 199).

When the supervisee describes their difficult experiences from psychotherapy in general, we lead them to define what is most difficult for them and to choose a concrete event representing this issue. Selecting the event and the specific difficult moment during that event enables the supervisee to feel their pain and suffering. We also invite the supervisee to come into contact with their body sensations related to the painful event, which enhances interoceptive awareness. Mindful awareness of their body sensations grounds the supervisee and enables full internal contact.

In this phase, useful questions are:

"What is most difficult for you in therapy with this client?"
"I would like to invite you to choose the event representing the most difficult part of the therapy with your client".
"What do you feel in your body when you think about this event (moment)?"

The supervisor asks this question with compassion. We have noticed that for supervisees this is relatively new, even challenging, when we direct their attention to themselves instead of to the client, especially if this focus involves compassionate inquiry into their experience of being with the client. Phenomenological compassionate inquiry encompasses the supervisor's care for the supervisee, how it is for them as a human being to be with the client in a difficult moment.

Realising and seeing themselves suffering may automatically evoke self-compassion in supervisees. In the subsequent three phases, we describe how the supervisor actively promotes self-compassion within the supervisee.

Phase 2: Promoting the supervisee's self-compassion

Promoting the supervisee's self-compassion for themselves, involves three sub-phases: 1) Leading the supervisee to look at themselves with loving eyes from a bird's eye perspective, 2) Promoting the supervisee's self-compassionate touch, and 3) Encouraging the supervisee's self-compassionate internal dialogue.

Leading the supervisee to look at themselves with loving eyes from a bird's perspective

In this step, the supervisor helps the supervisee to 1) Maintain a decentred position to their experience, and 2) Be a loving witness to their experience.

From the triangle of relationship to internal experience (Chapter 2, Figure 2.2), the supervisee can be merged, distant, or a loving witness in relation to their internal experience. The supervisor helps the supervisee to be a loving witness to their suffering instead of avoiding it or being overwhelmed by it. The loving witness position helps the supervisee to stay within the window of tolerance and enables them to be aware of their experience with acceptance and presence.

To facilitate the decentred perspective and witness stance, we lead the supervisee to look at their moment of suffering from a bird's eye view. To help the supervisee to be the compassionate and loving witness we suggest they look at themselves with loving eyes.

The supervisor might say:

"In your mind, go back to the therapy session, to that moment when it was the most difficult for you. Look at yourself with loving eyes from a bird's eye view. (short pause) What happens? or What do you notice?"

To promote the supervisee's compassion towards themselves, the supervisor might direct them to look at their body posture, which is often in a vulnerable position. Seeing themselves in a vulnerable body position may awaken self-compassion.

"When you observe yourself from a birds' perspective in what kind of posture is your body?"

To encourage the experience of self-compassion, the supervisor may also invite the supervisee to look at themselves as a person they deeply care about. The supervisor may say:

"Imagine that you are looking at a person that you deeply care about. (short pause) What happens?"

When the supervisee describes their experience, the supervisor may ask them what they feel towards themselves:

"While you are observing yourself from a bird's perspective with loving eyes, what do you feel towards yourself?"

Awareness of their feelings of kindness or love may strengthen the supervisee's self-compassion and internal contact. If the supervisee feels something different instead of compassion, with the help of this question, their attitude towards themselves comes into awareness and into the shared space with the supervisor.

Promoting the supervisee's compassionate self-touch

The supervisor may also propose that the supervisee gives themselves a compassionate touch while observing the critical psychotherapeutic event. Besides real touch, the supervisee may touch themselves in their imagination during the chosen critical moment.

The supervisor may say:

"If you agree, put your hand on your chest in a loving way". The supervisor says this in a gentle, kind, soft voice and may also put a hand on their own chest.

Or

"While observing yourself in the therapy room from a bird's perspective, would you like to come closer to yourself and touch yourself in a supportive way?"

The supervisor may also be more concrete in suggesting some specific supportive touch:

"While looking at yourself in the therapy room from a bird's perspective, would you come closer to yourself and put a hand on your shoulder?"

After a short while, the supervisor asks the supervisee: *"What do you notice?"* or *"What is happening?"* We do not leave the supervisee too long in their imagination.

Encouraging the supervisee's self-compassionate inner dialogue

If the supervisee is experiencing self-compassion, the supervisor may then initiate the self-compassionate inner dialogue. They may ask the supervisee what they would wish to tell themselves.

"Is there anything you would like to say to yourself?"

"What would you like to say to yourself from this compassionate state? What kind of words of support and love would you like to say? Be aware that your feeling of ____ (name their feeling they are struggling with) *is what we, psychotherapists, share".*

After the supervisee says their words of compassion to the vulnerable part of themselves, the supervisor may ask the vulnerable part to respond.

"How is it for you to hear those words of love and compassion?"

The inner dialogue can continue if needed until the supervisee experiences a loving inner connection and the experience of suffering is transformed. Insights regarding the therapy work can also arise in this phase.

Phase 3: Integration

In this last phase of integration, there are two sub-phases: 1) Connecting the supervisee's new self-compassionate state to the supervision problem, and 2) Reflection on the supervision process.

Connecting the supervisee's new self-compassionate state to the supervision problem

When the supervisee experiences self-compassion, the supervisor reminds them of the problem, they initially brought to supervision. In this way, they connect the supervisee's new self-compassionate self-state to the previous distressed state connected to the original supervision problem. Bearing in mind that this is supervision, this final stage is crucial. This self-compassion work with the supervisee needs to have both an implicit and explicit impact on their therapeutic work. By awakening a new resourceful state and connecting it to the supervision problem, the supervisee gains new insights into the therapeutic work: Their countertransference, the therapeutic relationship, client dynamics, or therapeutic interventions. By connecting the "new" resourceful state with the "old" distressed one, the supervisee's relational schema of being with the client is often transformed. We suggest that, in this way, we are encouraging memory reconsolidation (Ecker, 2018; Ecker et al., 2012; Lane et al., 2015). The supervisee may experience a *juxtaposition* between the initial relational schema related to distress and self-doubt with a new experience of self-compassion and safety. Such juxtaposition experiences are at the core of the memory reconsolidation process and may transform the initial dysfunctional relational schema. With the help of this process, supervisees, besides having new insights, enter the following therapy sessions transformed; their way of being with their clients changes, offering them presence and the possibility of contact in a therapeutic relationship. The present, mindful, and contactful way of being with the client is a vital facilitative therapeutic factor (Erskine, 2015; S. M. Geller & Greenberg, 2012; S. M. Geller, 2013; G. Žvelc & Žvelc, 2021).

To enhance the process of integration, the supervisor may invite the supervisee to imagine the next therapy session from their newly acquired state.

Reflection on the supervision process

The reflection phase offers time and space for debriefing the experience of self-compassion processing. The supervisor invites the supervisee to look at the whole supervision process from the presentation of the supervision question up to now. They invite the supervisee to reflect on how they experienced the whole process and the meaning the process has for them.

The supervisor might ask some of the following questions:

"If you look at the whole process as you have experienced it, how was it for you? What did the process bring to you? How might it help you for further work with this client? What is different now from the beginning of the session?"

While reflecting, supervisees often gain new insights connected to their psychotherapy work or elaborate on insights from earlier phases of self-compassion processing.

The reflection phase also includes meta-processing, a process inspired by Fosha's metatherapeutic processing (Fosha & Conceição, 2019; Fosha et al., 2019; Prenn & Fosha, 2017). It encompasses reflecting on the supervisee's positive experience during the supervision session. Supervisees become aware of the transformation of their experience, which occurred with the help of self-compassion processing. Supervisees may cherish a newly found loving and supportive attitude towards themselves, which they had temporarily lost but then regained during the self-compassion processing. The supervisor may also invite the supervisee to become aware of the relational aspect of the work.

"How was it for you to go through the process with your colleagues and me?"

The supervisor and supervision group members may also share their experience of the process and provide further juxtaposition experiences with their compassionate responses. Supervisees may be touched by the support they were given from the supervisor and the group and may show appreciation and gratitude.

Not forcing self-compassion

The supervisor does not force the supervisee to feel self-compassion. If the supervisee cannot bring compassion to themselves, the supervisor acknowledges, validates, and normalises that. The supervisor accepts the supervisee's current inability to be self-compassionate. The interruption of self-compassion has an important intrapsychic function and carries a significant story. The supervisor is compassionate towards the supervisee when they cannot find self-compassion. Maybe some deep wounds have been triggered within the supervisee, and personal therapy is needed to process their strong countertransference.

Vignettes of self-compassion processing

In the following two vignettes, we present self-compassion processing and the above-described phases. In each vignette a psychotherapist came to supervision impacted by the demanding therapy work, which was, in some parts, very stressful, causing them pain and suffering. In both vignettes, we turn the supervisee's attention inwards towards themselves and their vulnerability and then lead them towards self-compassion. Awakened self-care and kindness help them self-regulate and regain their internal balance, strength, and capacity to bond.

Vignette 1: Enhancing self-compassion in the supervision of complex trauma therapy: "I found my space in the body"

The supervisee Sandra, an experienced psychotherapist, presents the psychotherapy case with a client, a young woman in her twenties. The client was severely emotionally and physically abused since she was young and shows signs of complex trauma. The supervisee would like supervision to help her see the client's needs in the therapeutic relationship and what she is missing to give her.

Supervisee (speaking slowly):	*What am I missing? What does the client need, and I don't see it? I know she needs a lot of safe space. Maybe she needs a lot of time … but I as a therapist, I feel that I am not enough for her … . She is so traumatised. She is suffering so much. So … it's like maybe I am not safe enough for her.*
Supervisor:	(nodding).
Supervisee:	*The client has a strong transference towards me. She wants badly to be a good client. Sometimes she is also terrified of me; for instance, she freezes when I raise my hand. At such a moment, she sees me as a monster attacking her. She is afraid that she might lose control and kill me.*

While reading this, stop for a moment, and see how your body reacts. How would you feel if you were the therapist?

The supervisee is sitting upright and talking stoically. The supervisor hypothesises that this may be the supervisee's protection against feeling threatened and overwhelmed by the client's dysregulated and dissociated states.

Supervisor:	*Killing is a fantasy of traumatised children.*
Supervisee:	(nodding; her face starts to show suffering).
Supervisor:	*When I mentioned traumatised children, your eyes changed.*
Supervisee:	(nodding).
Supervisor (with compassionate expression and voice):	*Can you tell me what just happened inside of you?*

With phenomenological inquiry, the supervisor initiates mindful awareness of the supervisee's experience here and now.

Supervisee: *I see her as a very young child. And* (short silence; her eyes are getting wet, she briefly puts her hand on her chest) *I can feel her so much.* (The supervisee is talking with a shaking voice and starts crying gently.) *It was awful what happened to her. Nobody believed her. Nobody listened to her. She didn't have the chance to tell. She was so alone.*

The supervisee is very empathic, feeling the client's pain like it was her own, and based on *the model of the triangle of relationship to internal experience,* she is becoming merged with her experience. She is losing her decentred perspective. The client, in dysregulated emotional and physiological states, with a narrow window of tolerance, often influences the therapist's nervous system. It seems that here the supervisee's body has absorbed the client's trauma. The supervisee, Sandra, probably synchronised with the client's dysregulated physiology during therapy and is bringing this dysregulation into supervision. Maybe the supervisee is also reminded of herself in some way.

At this point, the supervisor feels that her own body tension is becoming stronger. This is a sign that she is synchronising with the supervisee's physiological dysregulation and a possible sign of a physiological parallel process. The supervisor's task is to stop this dysfunctional synchronisation and take the lead towards regulation. She initiates mindful observation of the supervisee's body and gives the supervisee time to breathe and explore her bodily reactions.

Supervisor: *Just breathe a little. What do you feel in your body now?*
Supervisee: *I feel tension. Here* (indicating her shoulders) (silence) ... *I can't breathe properly. My breathing is like ... I am breathing, and I am not breathing. And I feel very heavy shoulders, like somebody grabbed my shoulders and wanted to pull them back. You know, my client, as a child, was often violently grabbed by her shoulders.*

According to these body signs, the supervisee might now be at the edge of immobilisation. It is clear she is suffering. The supervisor decides to keep attention focused on the supervisee and decides to initiate self-compassion processing. She proceeds with phase 1, leading the supervisee to mindful awareness of the specific moment of her painful experience.

Supervisor (nodding):   *I have a suggestion. Are you willing to look at yourself and the client at your last session? And just take time to notice what is happening.* (talking in a kind and gentle voice).

The supervisee nods, meaning she is willing to do that. A few moments later:

Supervisee: *I am seeing two persons struggling … and both of us being very careful of each other … and I see myself wondering how afraid she is of me.*

The supervisor proceeds with the next phase of self-compassion processing, promoting the supervisee's self-compassion. In her following intervention, the supervisor combines subphases 2.1 and 2.2: Leading the supervisee to look at herself with loving eyes from a bird's perspective and promoting the supervisee's self-compassionate touch.

Supervisor: *Can we now look at you from outside, from a bird's perspective? A kind and gentle look at you. We can put a hand on your shoulder* (The supervisor's right-hand raises in the air, as if she is touching an imaginary Sandra). *Let this hand be warm and kind. And just notice what happens.*

The supervisor is using the expression we; she includes herself. In this way, her intervention is also relational, bringing her compassion to the supervisee, wishing that the supervisee feels that she is not alone and that someone is supporting her. This brings more safety to the supervisory relationship and improves the supervisee's self-compassion and regulation.

Working with trauma, also in the course of supervision, should include the body processes and awaken the body resources in the supervisee and the supervisor. With mindful awareness, breathing, words of compassion, and imaginative patting the supervisee's shoulder, the supervisor regulates the supervisee and also herself.

Supervisee: (Raises her left hand and mirrors the supervisor. Simultaneously, she is in her imagination touching her own shoulder during the last psychotherapy session. After a few seconds, she says): *It's ok, I am breathing. I can feel I am breathing* (Showing with her other hand her stomach and chest). *I feel warmth towards myself* (with a soft voice and compassionate expression).

The supervisee is regulating, returning to the window of tolerance, and recreating a safe, warm bond with herself. The supervisor also feels relief in her own body and feels touched by the supervisee's self-compassion and compassion towards the client. The supervisor looks into the supervisee's eyes and feels a moment of deep connection with the supervisee, which has a feeling of the spiritual; a meeting of two souls.

Supervisor:	*Somehow, through this conversation, I feel your good intention and connectedness to your client. I am touched.*
Supervisee (nodding, slightly wet eyes):	*I can feel your words.* (Indicating her chest).

The supervisee is moved, too. She is experiencing a state of self-compassion and contact within herself and with the supervisor.

Self-compassion transformed Sandra: Her physiology is regulated, her emotional experience is changed, and her cognitive functions are re-established. Now she can think more flexibly and get resourceful insights. The supervisor decides to initiate the third phase in self-compassion processing, integration. In the next intervention, she proceeds to subphase 3.1, connecting the supervisee's new compassionate state to the supervision problem and her previous schema of being with the client.

Supervisor (touching her chest):	*Can you now, from this state you are now experiencing, go back to your initial supervision question: What am I missing? Am I enough? Let's now think about this question.* (pause) *What do you get?*

The supervisor leads the supervisee back to the initial supervision question to facilitate the supervisee's own answer from her wisdom and knowledge. The supervisor directs the supervisee to hold this safe and self-compassionate state and at the same time to recall the initial supervision question related to confusion and threat. In this way, the supervisee is simultaneously aware of the previous dysregulated self-state and a new self-compassionate state. The supervisor is encouraging the "memory reconsolidation" process (Ecker et al., 2012). A new safe, regulated, self-compassionate state may provide a juxtaposition to the previous emotionally and physiologically dysregulated state and lead to its transformation.

Supervisee (short pause; in peaceful tone and rhythm):	*Yes, ... of course, I am enough.* (Touches her chest with one hand.) *But sometimes I think I am too much because relationships are so scary for her.*
Supervisor:	*What would help that you would not be too much, too scary for her?*
Supervisee:	*Let's explore that, yes.*

The supervisee and the supervisor explore the changes the supervisee can make in the therapeutic relationship to help the client feel safer. They discuss freeing up the space between the therapist and the client by changing their sitting positions, reducing the degree of eye contact, etc.

Supervisor: *I am noticing that we are not talking about more but less.*
Supervisee: *Yes, exactly. I am calmer now.*
Supervisor: *So now we are approaching the end .... Let's debrief a little.* (Both of them take a deep breath a few times) *Remember the beginning of the supervision and your motivation to present this case. You were asking, what is missing, I am not enough, and then, take a look at the whole session which followed. Can you reflect on all that we did?*

The supervisor initiates the last phase of self-compassion processing, subphase 3.2, reflection on the supervision process.

Supervisee: *When I came here, I felt I was just like lost in space* (showing confused circles with hands). *I wasn't in contact with the earth. Now I feel I am more here. With so many things, my inner world was just stuck* (hands doing short, cutting movements). *Her story, her images, my images, what happened to her .... And now ... there's a space in my body. And it is interesting. Before, I was like: Where should I put all this?!? I have to do something with this!* (Her voice becomes, for a moment, louder and more critical.). *And I thought I should do more in therapy with her.* (smiling). *Yes.*
Supervisor: *And now you feel like you have space.*
Supervisee: *And I should give her that space, yes.*

The supervisee reflects on her transition from being overwhelmed and stuck to a state of groundedness and presence. Her emotional and physiological state was endangered and dysregulated in response to the client's reactions and her own self-imposed pressure to be sufficient for the client. Self-compassion processing in the course of supervision helped her regain supportive contact with herself, ground herself, and feel safer. She successfully differentiated between herself and the client. Metaphorically speaking, before, the client's trauma was absorbed in the supervisee's body, taking away her own space, and now, in supervision, the supervisee found a space in her body. In the next psychotherapy session, she can offer the client this new present state of being. Her groundedness and presence will also direct her decisions regarding psychotherapy work. In addition to the benefit for psychotherapy with the client, the self-compassion process also benefitted the welfare of the supervisee. It nurtured the supervisee, balanced her body and sense of self, and regained her sense of worth as a psychotherapist.

Vignette 2: The therapist regains her pride and self-support after facing the client's complaints

In vignette 2, we present an excerpt from the self-compassion processing with the supervisee Mary who was finding her work with a particular couple very stressful.

Supervisee: *I have in mind a couple I have been working with for some time. Both partners are so wounded. There is such reactivity between them, and I often feel: "Have we done anything at all? What will come out of this? Will anything come out of it?" Despite that, I see they have been with me for more than a year and that there are steps forward; they go further now. But these steps are so small that I am personally sometimes in despair.*

The therapist being in despair is a marker for the initiation of self-compassion processing.

Supervisor: *Mary, what is it that is most difficult above all else?*

The supervisor wants to narrow the problem and make it more specific.

Supervisee: *Maybe this part; they, especially the wife, complain that nothing we are doing makes any difference.*

When Mary shares these words, the supervisor feels like something has hit her in the chest. She hypothesises it must hurt Mary to hear these words. The supervisor discloses her bodily response:

Supervisor (firmly, decisively,   *I felt a sharp pain when you told me that.* (Short
puts her hand on her chest):   pause). *Does she exactly say this in the session?*
Supervisee: *Yes. Several times.*
Supervisor (with a   *Can you recall a part of the session, a specific*
compassionate   *moment, which was the most difficult for you,*
expression on her face):   *when she complained?*

The supervisor initiates phase 1 of self-compassion processing: Leading the supervisee to mindful awareness of her painful experience.

Supervisee: *Yes.*
Supervisor: *Can you describe it?*
Supervisee: *It did not happen just once; it happened several times, and usually after one of them has managed to dive more into the depths. And then, for her, this is my interpretation, it was somehow unsafe to see this depth, even a relatively small amount. And feeling the pain in herself or her partner. And then this sentence came out of her. And not just words; she physically closes herself off totally.* (The supervisee shows with her hands, as if putting up a wall in front of her chest and stomach.)

The supervisee has not shared a specific moment. This may be a sign of self-protection. She is paying attention to the client and interpreting her dynamics. The supervisor wants to direct the supervisee's attention to herself. She aims to lead the supervisee to an embodied awareness of how it is for her with this client and then bring self-support through kindness and self-compassion.

Supervisees are usually accustomed to talking and caring about their clients; it is more difficult for them to turn to themselves and care for themselves. Here, the supervisor wishes to give space and attention to the supervisee. She wants to lead the supervisee to be mindfully aware of a specific moment of suffering; that's why she comes back with the question:

Supervisor: *Can you choose a specific moment when the client physically closed herself off?*

Supervisee: *She closes down; the physiognomy of her face changes at once. Not just her face but her whole body. An impenetrable block.* (The supervisee shows with her hands a wall in front of her chest and stomach). *Intensely cold, her mouth set in one line, and then these words pour out that there is no point in coming to therapy, she does not know what she is doing here, nothing moves forward.*

Supervisor: *Ok, I understand. This woman shuts herself* off (showing with her hands the wall in front of her) *and* says *there is no point.*

Supervisee: *Yes.*

The supervisee recalls the concrete event, and the supervisor moves to the second phase of self-compassion processing, promoting the supervisee's self-compassion. The following intervention presents subphase 2.1, leading the supervisee to look at herself with loving eyes from outside, from a bird's perspective.

Supervisor: *Do you agree to continue further with this, and now, looking down from a bird's perspective, look at yourself and your clients, the wife and her husband. You can have your eyes open or closed, as you prefer.*
        Pause.
        And now, from this bird's perspective, look at yourself with a loving attitude. And let me know what you see.

Supervisee: *Besides this sudden change in the wife, I also freeze.*

While the supervisee is talking, the supervisor takes a few deep breaths. She needs to breathe to counteract the pressure in her chest, which is rising inside her. The rising pressure in her chest may indicate significant physiological changes in the supervisee.

Supervisor: *Yes, you are seeing how you freeze.*
Supervisee: *Although I am looking down from a bird's perspective, I feel this freezing, here, in my chest.* (With her hand making circles in the chest area.)
Supervisor: *Ah, yes, that means it is powerful. It is not only there during therapy but also here and now.*
Supervisee: *Yes.*

Mary's freezing while observing herself indicates that she is losing her decentred position and merging with her experience, triggered by remembering the therapy session. Her physiological state is dysregulated, and the supervisor decides to regulate the supervisee here and now with the help of self-compassionate touch (Subphase 2.2).

Supervisor: *You feel it in your chest, right?*
Supervisee: *Yes, in my chest.*
Supervisor: *Can you put one hand on your chest, on your heart, in a gentle, compassionate way?*
Supervisee (closed eyes): *I'll put both hands on my chest. I need both hands, not just one.*
Supervisor: *Yes, that's fine.* (Silence. The supervisor has an attentive, compassionate look and breathes a little more deeply.)
Supervisee: *When I look from above, I feel some pride. I feel that this freezing in my chest is acting like a block and is helping me; I do not take all of these harsh words upon myself.*
Supervisor: *That's right. It is some kind of protection, isn't it?*
Supervisee: *Yes, when I look at myself from above, I see that I can, I have this ability, to see that these accusations are not all my fault.*
Supervisor (nodding):   *Yes, that's right.*
Supervisee: *My part in all these complaints is relatively small, even though whenever she starts to complain, it shakes me, but I don't let all her criticism affect me.*

The supervisee gains a significant insight that the freezing block in her chest protects her from the wife's critical attacks. The supervisee also changes her perception of herself, that it is not all her fault for what the client is accusing her.

Supervisor: *I see. This is an important insight.*
Supervisee: *Yes.*

Supervisor: *Do you agree that we come back to the therapy session, and you look with loving eyes at yourself from a bird's perspective? Tell me, what body posture do you have when you look at yourself?*

The supervisor guides the supervisee into seeing her posture in the therapy session. If the supervisee sees her body posture in a vulnerable position, that may open the supervisee to feeling her pain and, subsequently, self-compassion.

Supervisee:	*The wife attacks me, and I lean back. When I lean back, the distance between us is bigger than before.*
Supervisor (putting a hand on her chest):	*Ok, you see that you are leaning back. Is there anything else you see?*
Supervisee (indicating her chest):	*No, just the block is here.*

It seems that the supervisee is still merged with her experience. In the next intervention, the supervisor again encourages Mary to look at herself from a bird's perspective to promote a decentred perspective. She wishes the supervisee to observe how her body looks from the outside perspective instead of focusing on her sensations within. In this way, we help her differentiate between the observing self and her experience.

Supervisor: *From a bird's perspective, is there perhaps anything else you can see from the outside?*
  Silence.
Supervisee: *No. Perhaps a little, yes. Stiffness of the body. Mostly in this part* (indicating her chest), *and my knees and legs below the knees are tight.*
Supervisor: *Mary, can we say, when we are watching you in that difficult moment, such moments are difficult; could we say you are suffering?*

The supervisor uses the plural – we to convey support and togetherness, that the supervisee is not alone. She chooses the word suffering to point the supervisee towards meeting her pain. The supervisor's look is very compassionate.

Supervisee:	*I would not use this word, but it is definitely not good.*
Supervisor (feeling emotional pain inside, with a compassionate expression in her eyes and face):	*Ok, so we can say it is definitely not good.*
Supervisee:	*Yes.*

Supervisor (with gentle, compassionate voice, slow pace):	*What do you, in this moment, while you are observing yourself, feel towards yourself?*

This question can help the supervisee to feel and express compassion towards herself.

Supervisee (hands on her chest):	*While observing, I feel compassion. I see that down there, in the therapy room, I strive to do my best. I am telling myself: "You are doing well". In my observing eyes, I have the same look as when I watch one of my kids in a difficult situation. And I am saying: "Bravo". (She raises her fist, showing her strength. Her face and voice soften.)*

While observing her pain from a decentred position, the supervisee spontaneously starts an internal self-compassionate dialogue (subphase 2.3), supporting herself by telling herself she is doing well. She encourages and empowers herself. Before, she was blocked, whereas now her newly established strength counteracts immobilisation.

The supervisor feels appreciation for the supervisee's process. On the other hand, inside her body, she still feels emotional pain. She may, through physiological synchronisation, be sensing Mary's pain, which is hidden somewhere deeper. The supervisor now initiates subphase 2.2, promoting the supervisee's self-compassionate touch.

Supervisor:	*Would you like to touch yourself in some way? Perhaps give yourself a pat on your shoulder?*
Supervisee (with energy and enthusiasm):	*I would go there and hug myself and say to myself: "You are doing fine; this is difficult to endure, super!"*
Supervisor (the sparkle in her eyes, wide gentle smile):	*Ok, let's do that.*
Supervisee (Hugs herself in reality and in her mind's eye during the therapy session. Then she starts gently crying.):	*This moves me a lot.*

The supervisee comes into contact with her pain and becomes profoundly compassionate to herself. The supervisor is also very touched. Her eyes are slightly wet and sparkling. She is nodding. She is present.

Supervisor (with one hand on her chest):	*This is a good sign.*

Supervisee:	(visibly exhales with the sound 'hu', like she is exhaling all the burden from working with that couple).
	Silence.
Supervisor:	*Just allow yourself … . this is a significant moment; you came into touch with yourself.*

The supervisee's state significantly changed from when she initially presented the problem; now, she is kind and supportive towards herself, open and in contact with herself and the supervisor. The relational schema of being with the client at the beginning of the session consisted of despair and a feeling of threat, resulting in a block, bodily felt in the chest, and tight legs. Through self-compassion processing, the supervisee regained her pride, strength, self-support, and kindness to herself. With the help of this change, she can lead the next therapy session more flexibly instead of withdrawing. Being in contact with herself, she could now initiate an alliance rupture repair and communicate with the clients about her and their experience; if needed, she may set some boundaries.

Self-compassion processing was also beneficial for the supervisee as a person. The block she experienced was draining her energy. By self-compassion processing, she transformed this block into strength and care.

Chapter 12

Self-care and prevention of burnout in mindfulness- and compassion-oriented supervision

In this chapter, we present how supervision, by promoting mindful aware-ness, self-compassion, and physiological regulation, encourages the super-visee's self-care and prevents burnout. Working with clients is often demanding and stressful and may trigger intense emotions and physiological reactions that therapists experience during therapy sessions or outside their work. Often therapists lack the self-permission to attend to themselves and take care of themselves during psychotherapy sessions. Our role as supervi-sors is to direct them and show them how to care for themselves. In this chapter, we present a supervision model called MANER, which shows how supervision by promoting mindful awareness, self-compassion and physio-logical regulation encourages the supervisee's self-care. We are especially interested in developing the therapist's ability to track mindfully, moment-to-moment, their body/physiological responses during supervision and psycho-therapy sessions, and be kind to themselves. Through three vignettes from supervisory sessions, we demonstrate how regulation with the help of mindfulness and self-compassion is a significant factor in self-care and pre-venting burnout.

Many self-care activities contribute to the welfare of therapists. Some activities can be implemented outside the psychotherapy session in the su-pervisee's daily life, and some within the therapy session (see Figure 12.1). Outside the therapy session, therapists can take care of themselves and strengthen resilience by enhancing social connections. Socialising with friends, spouses, children, relatives, and others is an important way of self-care that promotes the satisfaction of relational needs (Erskine, 2015). Satisfaction of relational needs is related to better well-being, higher satis-faction with life, and self-compassion (G. Žvelc et al., 2020). Essential self-care activities are also related to play, creativity, having meaningful hobbies, sports, and recreation. Another area we find particularly helpful for promoting self-care is meditation practice. We may advise therapists to learn different meditation practices. Mindfulness and self-compassion meditations are par-ticularly congruent with our approach as they may strengthen the therapist's capacity for mindful awareness and self-compassion during the psychotherapy

DOI: 10.4324/9781003194118-15

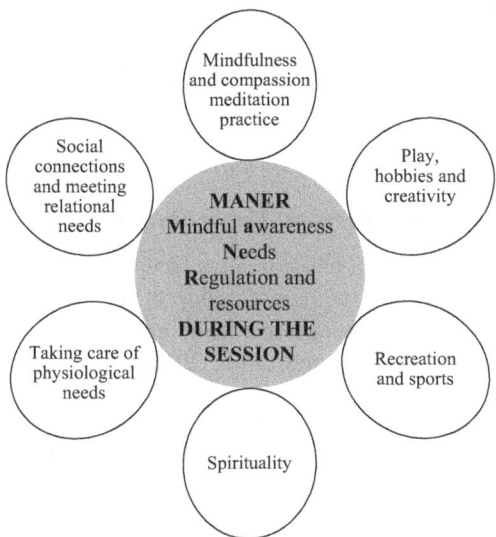

Figure 12.1 The flower of self-care.

session. However, some therapists prefer contemplative practices related to body awareness and mindful movements, such as tai-chi or yoga. Research shows that a therapist's or counsellor's mindfulness meditation practice reduces stress or prevents burnout (Felton et al., 2015; Mohammed et al., 2018; Shapiro et al., 2007; Yip et al., 2017). For some therapists, important resources are spirituality-related activities, which help supervisees self-regulate and provide a sense of meaning in life.

It is also essential that therapists take care of their basic physiological needs like drinking enough water, eating regular meals, having a healthy diet, getting sufficient sleep, and physical movement. Healthcare workers are more prone to stress reactions when their physiological and psychological needs are left unsatisfied. Above all, it is important that therapists are gentle and kind to themselves. If therapists take care of the above-mentioned needs, they will have a better capacity for performing psychotherapy and implementing self-care during the therapy session.

This chapter focuses on how supervision models and teaches supervisees to provide self-care within the therapy session and prevents their emotional distress. We developed the supervision model MANER, which shows how we direct supervisees to the significance of mindful awareness, needs, regulation, and resources within the supervision and therapy session. In the next sub-chapter, we introduce both the research and the theoretical basis of the MANER model.

Mindful awareness and compassion as protective factors for psychotherapists

Mindfulness and self-compassion are associated with self-care and prevention of burnout by facilitating stress regulation and the development of positive, secure inner attachment.

Mindfulness as a protective factor in the prevention of burnout

Research shows that mindful capacity positively connects to vitality and well-being among mental health practitioners (Martin-Cuellar et al., 2021) and that a mindfulness meditation practice prevents burnout among therapists and counsellors (Felton et al., 2015; Mohammed et al., 2018; Shapiro et al., 2007; Yip et al., 2017).

Mindful awareness enables emotional regulation (Farb et al., 2012; Goldin & Gross, 2010; Hayes & Feldman, 2004; Price & Hooven, 2018; Teper et al., 2013; Vago & Silbersweig, 2012). A systematic review, which shows the association between emotional regulation and burnout among doctors, found that mindfulness is a significant regulation strategy for reducing burnout (Jackson-Koku & Grime, 2019). Studies show that burnout is related to emotional suppression and lower cognitive reappraisal (Chalikkandy et al., 2022; Martín-Brufau et al., 2020), which may explain the beneficial effects of mindfulness. Mindfulness enables people to stay in contact with emotions instead of suppressing them, which is an important regulation strategy.

Mindful awareness enables self-care and burnout prevention because it also helps the psychotherapist take a decentred position to their experience and distinguish between themselves and the client. Research shows that psychotherapists with weaker differentiation between themselves and clients are more prone to experience empathic distress (Uršič & Žvelc, 2017) and that emotionally overinvolved psychotherapists experience significantly higher levels of emotional exhaustion (Lee et al., 2011). The decentred position prevents merging and over-involvement. It allows the optimal and balanced distance between the client and the therapist's experience. This helps the therapist to stop the dysfunctional synchronisation with the client and prevent them from absorbing their stress.

Compassion and prevention of burnout

For psychotherapists, it is essential that they are empathic to their clients. However, the constant feeling of others' pain and suffering may lead to empathic distress and burnout (Klimecki et al., 2013). We tend to synchronise with others' physiological states (Palumbo et al., 2017) and emotional expressions (Hatfield et al., 2014) and absorb their stress. When we are empathic with the person in pain, "our brain will show activation of similar circuits as the brain of the person with whom we are empathising" (Hofmeyer et al., 2020, p. 3).

Compassion, in contrast to empathy, prevents burnout (Klimecki et al., 2013). Research shows that training in empathic resonance increases negative affect and that subsequent compassion training reverses the increase of negative affect (Klimecki et al., 2013). The research also shows that different brain circuits activate when feeling empathic as opposed to when being compassionate. When empathic, there is an activation of the brain networks playing a crucial role in empathy for pain, self-experienced pain, and negative affect (Klimecki et al., 2013). When we are compassionate, the brain networks connected to positive affect, reward, and affiliation activate (Klimecki et al., 2013). Compassion goes beyond empathy as it offers a resonating response to a person in pain and suffering and requires the distinction between the self and the other (Erskine, 2020). When we feel compassion, we respond to the client's pain by experiencing corresponding positive affect related to the care and well-being of another person. Such positive affective states are positively related to the therapist's well-being and prevent empathic distress.

Self-compassion: The essential component of self-care

Self-compassion of mental health professionals is significantly related to their well-being and is negatively connected to stress and burnout (Atkinson et al., 2017; Eriksson et al., 2018; Kastelic et al., 2022; Kotera et al., 2021; Richardson et al., 2020; Voon et al., 2021).

Therapists who are highly critical of themselves and their work are more vulnerable to burnout (Richardson et al., 2020). Self-compassion helps to reduce self-criticism and shame (Gilbert & Procter, 2006; Sedighimornani et al., 2019) and is an effective mediator between self-criticism and burnout (Richardson et al., 2020).

Self-compassion promotes emotional regulation, which is a significant change factor contributing to mental health (Barlow et al., 2017; Bates et al., 2021; Diedrich et al., 2016; Finlay-Jones, 2017; Inwood & Ferrari, 2018; Scoglio et al., 2015; Vettese et al., 2011). Self-compassion also stimulates a secure attachment to ourselves, which raises feelings of safety.

Neurobiological research indicates that self-compassion reduces defensiveness by deactivating the threat system and raises safety by activating the caregiving system (Arch et al., 2014; Rockliff et al., 2008). Soothing touch raises oxytocin levels and reduces cortisol response to stress (Dreisoerner et al., 2021; Uvnäs-Moberg et al., 2014). Self-compassionate training reduces sympathetic alpha-amylase response and modulates heart-rate variability response (HRV) (Arch et al., 2014). Young adults with higher dispositional self-compassion show lower stress-induced reactivity of salivary alpha-amylase (sAA), a marker of sympathetic nervous system activation (Breines et al., 2015). In individuals with higher social safeness and self-compassion, compassion-focused imagery (an imagination that someone is compassionate towards yourself) was related to an increase in HRV and a decrease in cortisol levels (Rockliff et al., 2008).

There is consistent evidence regarding the positive role of mindfulness and self-compassion in the well-being of mental health practitioners and the prevention of stress and burnout. However, to our knowledge, contemporary research has not yet explored the therapist's mindful awareness or self-compassion during psychotherapy sessions. We propose further research to explore the connection between the therapist's mindful awareness and self-compassion during therapy sessions with other variables such as job satisfaction, emotional distress, burnout, and psychotherapy outcome variables.

Our primary suggestion is for the therapist to be mindfully aware, moment to moment, of their body and physiological state during each therapy session (G. Žvelc & Žvelc, 2021). As Safran and Muran (2000) suggest, the therapist's *mindfulness in action* is needed during the therapy session. A therapist, who is mindfully aware of their physiological arousal, will be able to regulate it.

Emotional and physiological regulation as a protective factor for the psychotherapist's health and well-being

Research among healthcare practitioners shows that using emotional regulation strategies negatively correlates with burnout (Chalikkandy et al., 2022; Jackson-Koku & Grime, 2019; Martín-Brufau et al., 2020). Clinical practice and research data support the importance of regulation with mindfulness and self-compassion as a significant self-care factor in the prevention of burnout (Coaston, 2017; Eriksson et al., 2018; Kotera et al., 2021; Mantelou & Karakasidou, 2019; Martin-Cuellar et al., 2021; Yip et al., 2017; G. Žvelc & Žvelc, 2021).

In our supervision practice, we notice that supervisees who "bring" into supervision dysregulated emotional and physiological states from their psychotherapy work and who were previously unaware of them often report sleep disturbances, tiredness, digestive problems, different kinds of pain in the body, fibromyalgia, and other symptoms. We suggest that supervisees who lose mindful awareness and lack physiological regulation during therapy sessions are more prone to emotional distress and burnout. We propose that burnout is connected to what Levine (2018) calls *autonomic dysregulation syndrome*. Autonomic dysregulation syndrome is related to symptoms such as body tension and pain, chronic fatigue, irritable bowel syndrome, gastric reflux, digestive problems, certain cardiac arrhythmias, low or high blood pressure, fibromyalgia, migraines, and others. Levine (2018) argues that the syndrome is a stress-related disorder of regulation. The dysregulation of the autonomous nervous system plays a primary part in the development of that syndrome. Our survival reactions of fight, flight, and freeze, are designed to be temporary and turn off when the threat is over. With its mobilisation and immobilisation responses, prolonged stress becomes toxic and affects health (Yaribeygi et al., 2017). "Opportunity for treatment lies in interventions that reestablish organismic self-regulation" (Levine, 2018, p. 22). We can paraphrase this and say that the opportunity for prevention of burnout lies in the physiological and emotional regulation of the psychotherapist during the psychotherapy session and in daily life.

Physiological synchrony and stress contagiousness in psychotherapy

The psychotherapy process is an intersubjective process in which the therapist influences the client, and the client influences the therapist. Their emotional and physiological states are contagious (Hatfield et al., 2014; Rothschild, 2006; G. Žvelc & Žvelc, 2021). The physiological synchrony research into the psychotherapy relationship shows that the physiology of the therapist synchronises with the client's physiology and vice versa (Bar-Kalifa et al., 2019; Kleinbub, 2017; Kleinbub et al., 2020; Marci & Orr, 2006; Palmieri et al., 2018; Tschacher & Meier, 2019). This means that the therapist's body responds to the client's body and vice versa (Rothschild, 2006; G. Žvelc & Žvelc, 2021). Therapists can thus easily "catch" the physiological stress of the clients (Buchanan et al., 2012), which is a health risk for mental health professionals.

These significant findings suggest that the therapist's body, when working with clients, is exposed to the dysregulated ANS of their clients and reacts to it with synchronisation. This means that when we work with clients with dysregulated physiology, for instance, with traumatised clients, we are vulnerable to synchronising with these dysregulated physiological states and staying within dysregulation. When the therapist does not recognise that they synchronise with the client's dysregulated state and stay within this dysregulation, they are prone to destabilise their health and develop empathic distress and burnout.

The fundamental key in the therapy situation is for the therapist to recognise their synchronisation with the dysregulated physiological states of the client and regulate their own physiology (G. Žvelc & Žvelc, 2021).

Functional and dysfunctional physiological synchrony

We propose two kinds of physiological synchrony in psychotherapy and supervision: 1) Functional, which enables compassion and a good alliance, and is related to a regulated response, and 2) Dysfunctional, which leads to dysregulated physiological states (see Chapter 4). We propose that prolonged dysfunctional synchronisation negatively impacts the quality of the therapeutic process and affects the therapist's well-being and health. Our division of physiological synchrony is based on the research of Helm et al. (2014) on *morphostatic* and *morphogenic* physiological synchrony, where morphostatic would correspond to functional and morphogenic to dysfunctional synchrony.

Functional synchrony refers to a process of synchronisation with another person's physiology when they are within or close to regulated physiological states. This means that when another person is within the window of tolerance with optimal ANS arousal, this positively impacts the first person's nervous system. Functional synchrony enables attunement and compassion, gives the client a feeling that they are deeply understood, and promotes a good therapeutic relationship.

Dysfunctional synchronisation happens when we are synchronising with another person's physiology, when they are in a dysregulated physiological state, outside the window of tolerance. Because of this, we may also experience physiological dysregulation, which shows in either hyper- or hypoarousal. Based on our supervision experience, the therapist, synchronising in this dysfunctional way, is often unaware of this dysfunctional synchronisation and stays for longer than is either healthy or necessary in those defensive physiological states. This makes them more prone to develop empathic distress, autonomic dysregulation syndrome, and burnout. The solution we strongly recommend is that the therapist becomes mindfully aware that they are synchronising with dysregulated physiology of the client, stop this dysfunctional synchronisation, regulate themselves, and lead the client towards regulation (G. Žvelc & Žvelc, 2021). In the supervision process, we teach therapists through modelling how to develop these skills that promote optimal *physiological attunement* (see Chapter 9). In our previous work, we wrote that physiological attunement is "sensing the physiological arousal of the client and providing the corresponding response" (G. Žvelc & Žvelc, 2021, p. 128). The corresponding adaptive response is related to physiological synchronisation with the client when their physiological state is regulated. This means that both the therapist and the client will be in the optimal arousal zone. When the client's ANS is dysregulated, in a hyper- or hypoarousal state, the therapist's corresponding response stops the physiological synchronisation and provides physiological regulation for themselves and the client. In this case, the therapist may feel distress related to the client; however, they regulate themselves and lead the client towards regulation (see Chapters 4 and 9).

When therapists are empathic towards their clients, but without a clear sense of themselves and their boundaries, they are more prone to empathic distress and burnout (Hofmeyer et al., 2020; Singer & Klimecki, 2014; Uršič & Žvelc, 2017). Being merged with the client's emotional and physiological states can negatively affect the therapist's physiological system, further affecting the therapist's emotional processes, perception, and cognitive functions. We strongly agree with Rothschild (2006), saying that for the sake of the therapist's well-being, "she needs to be able to find ways to balance her empathetic engagement [and] regulate her ANS arousal" (p. 3). Based on research and our clinical experiences as therapists and supervisors, we suggest that the state of the therapist's regulated physiological system during the therapy is both a crucial psychotherapy factor and a factor that prevents job-related stress (G. Žvelc & Žvelc, 2021). If the therapist's arousal is within the window of tolerance, they are aware of their boundaries, can think clearly (Ogden et al., 2006; Rothschild, 2006), and can be optimally physiologically attuned.

Last but not least, we want to emphasise that all the recommended methods and interventions in supervision intended for the practitioner's self-care are effective only where there is a good supervision alliance. A better supervisory relationship negatively predicts burnout symptoms among health professionals (Hiebler-Ragger et al., 2021).

MANER: A supervision model for prevention and self-care

In various chapters of this book, we have provided different methods for enhancing mindful awareness, compassion, and emotional and physiological regulation. The MANER model synthesises this knowledge and emphasises its use for the therapist's self-care and stress prevention.

We propose the following strategies for the prevention of burnout and self-care, linked to the acronym MANER (see Figure 12.1):

- MA- mindful awareness of body and physiological states
- NE- recognition of needs
- R- regulation and building resources.

The MANER model is based on the mindful embodiment of the professional, where our physiological responses are the compass for our protection and self-care. Knowing and listening to the body is a royal road to our well-being.

Based on the MANER model, the supervisor encourages the supervisee to be mindfully aware of their body, physiological states, and needs during the therapy and supervision sessions. They learn to regulate themselves when needed and activate their resources. One of the significant resources is self-compassion.

We receive consistent feedback from our supervisees that by following these suggestions (see Box 12.1), their sessions become more manageable, and they are not so tired afterward. If therapists are mindfully aware of their body and physiological state, they are taking a decentred perspective at that moment. This perspective helps them differentiate between themselves and their experience and between themselves and the client. The differentiation from the clients allows the therapist not to be caught by and sucked into the resonance with the client's dysregulated nervous system.

Some therapists think good therapy is about giving all of themselves to a client; but in doing this, they lose their boundaries and sense of self. They ignore their capacity to self-regulate and care for themselves. Emotional overinvolvement is linked to emotional exhaustion (Lee et al., 2011).

Mindful awareness informs us about the condition of our emotional and physiological states, and from an awareness that our states are dysregulated,

---

Box 12.1   Suggestions for self-care during the psychotherapy session

Based on the MANER model, we would advise you, whether a psychotherapist or other mental health professional, to take care of yourself in the following ways:

- Be mindfully aware of your body during the psychotherapy session.
- Be mindfully aware of the signs which indicate that you are in hyperarousal or hypoarousal within the psychotherapy session.
- Be aware of what it is your need in that particular moment in the psychotherapy session.
- When needed, take a mindful pause for awareness and regulation of yourself and the client. Go with the pace that you both can manage.
- Be gentle, kind, and compassionate to yourself during the psychotherapy session.

---

we can self-regulate. Mindful awareness promotes regulation by itself. It enables us to be aware of our body's adaptive action tendencies; what the body needs and would like to do. We may become aware that our body would like to breathe (we may previously have stopped breathing); maybe it tells us that our body wants to move. We know a therapist who, to be fully "present" for the client, did not allow herself to move. Consequently, she lost all sense of her legs and could not feel them anymore. She was not aware of her im-mobilisation response. At the end of the session, when she went to stand up, she fell and broke her leg.

Unfortunately, from our training and supervision experience, we have seen how therapists often miss the signs when they or their clients are dysregu-lated. Because of this, we developed the MANER model and emphasise the saying: "therapist first" (G. Žvelc & Žvelc, 2021), meaning that therapists should primarily be mindfully aware of their own physiological states. Only after first regulating themselves, do they then help their clients towards reg-ulation. Box 12.2 presents further directions for therapists to enhance mindful awareness during the therapy session.

Supervision vignettes: Learning in supervision how to provide self-care during a psychotherapy session

All the vignettes in the previous chapters of this book are linked to the su-pervisee's self-care and stress prevention. In most of those vignettes, we were working with the supervisee's disturbing countertransference, regulating and transforming their physiological and emotional states, mostly with the help of

---

Box 12.2   Mindful awareness during the session: Directions for psychotherapists

During the therapy session, bring awareness to your body. Follow the intentions of your body; they will help you to take care of yourself and regulate yourself.

If you go beyond the boundaries of the window of tolerance, if you are in hyper- or hypo-arousal, then the client is also likely to be dysregulated.

When you are mindfully aware of your dysregulated state, regulate yourself (for instance, by breathing) and gently invite the client to become mindfully aware of their states. If they are in dysregulated states, take time for regulation. In the meantime, when you help the client to regulate, you will also regulate yourself.

This is the same as the situation in an aeroplane; when there is not enough oxygen, we first have to put the mask on our own mouth, and then we will be able to put the mask on the child (the client).

---

mindful awareness and self-compassion. You can read all those vignettes again and look at them through the eyes of self-care for the supervisee.

The following three supervision vignettes show stress prevention and self-care work using the MANER model. In the first vignette, we promote, with the help of mindful awareness, the therapist's embodied self-protective strategies (as setting the self-boundary). In the second vignette, we show how the supervisee, with the help of mindful awareness and self-compassion, finds her strength for working with a very passive client. In the third vignette, we show how through mindful awareness of her body, the supervisee discovers her anger towards the client as her resource for setting boundaries.

Vignette 1: "I feel protected and nurtured": Exploring embodied self-care strategies

The supervisee Betty comes to the supervision session with the complaint that she feels her clients drain her and would like to do something regarding this. She has in mind the psychotherapy with one client, after which she feels particularly exhausted. In recent years she developed the symptoms of fibromyalgia. The previous month she had a bad relapse and started asking herself if the work with that client, with severely dysregulated physiology, might worsen her state. She already uses some mindfulness and self-compassion techniques to help herself regulate while she is alone. In the presented supervision session, we realised that she lacks the permission and embodied strategies for regulating and taking care of herself in therapeutic relationships. In this session, we explore what happens in her body while working with this client. Working with her and other supervisees with autonomic dysregulation syndrome (Levine, 2018), we realised that bottom-up supervision is vitally important. Working only on the cognitive understanding of therapy processes is not enough and cannot change the supervisee's body responses during the therapy session.

The supervisor asks Betty to recall the last therapy session with that particular client. While she recalls the session, the supervisor leads Betty to mindful awareness of her body. This is the first step of MANER - MA: Mindful awareness of the body and physiological states.

Supervisor: Betty, what are you experiencing in your body now?

Betty answers that she is becoming aware that she is nervous and agitated. She feels this all over her body, but mainly in her chest. Her heart is beating faster. These are signs of sympathetic activation and dysregulation of her ANS. She is in hyperarousal. The other group member Sara then asks her to show the body posture representing how she relates to this client in the therapy. Betty opens and expands her hands widely. She looks as if she would give everything from herself to the client. Her chest is open, completely uncovered. For the supervisor, Betty's chest seems too vulnerable in that open position, and the supervisor feels an inner need to gently cross her hands on her own chest.

Supervisor:	*What do you feel in your body while you open your hands like that?* (step MA: Mindful awareness of the body and physiological states)
Supervisee Betty:	*I feel unprotected. I don't feel well in that posture. Like I am giving all of myself to the client. I feel anxious.*
Supervisee Sara, the other group member:	*Oh, I would feel terrible like that. Like I can be shot directly in my heart. Or, like I will be crucified.*
Supervisor to Betty:	*Which movement, or posture, would make you feel more protected? Notice what your body would like to do.*

The supervisor is going further to the next step, NE: The recognition of needs.

Betty moves her hands a little more closely to each other. Her position still stays quite open. The supervisor mirrors the position and doesn't feel comfortable in it.

Supervisor:	*How do you feel in this position?* (step MA: Mindful awareness of the body and physiological states)
Supervisee Betty:	*A little better … but still upset, anxious …*

Supervisor:	*How would it be for you to put your hands like this?* (Supervisor follows her own body intentions and gently, compassionately crosses her hands over her own chest.)

Betty mirrors it, as well as the other member of the group. Betty starts rocking herself; she is gentle to herself, providing nurturing and self-regulation (step R: Regulation and building resources). Soon she starts to cry. It looks like it is a cry of relief.

Supervisee Betty	*It feels so good. I feel protected and nurtured. I forgot*
(after a short time):	*that this is possible ... is this also possible in therapy? Good .... But ... can I be like that with clients? I have a feeling if I am like that, that I don't give them enough.*

Betty regulates herself with this change of body posture and compassionate self-nurturing. She comes to an embodied place of safety. She actively experimented with the body position of nurturance and protection and found a resource in this body position. She could use this position in therapy or imagine herself being in this position while being with the client. After some time, her old script activated, based on a dysfunctional relational schema, that she should give all of herself to others, take care of them, and not pay attention to herself. The supervisor gave her "permission" to take care of herself during the therapy sessions. After that, they all, including the other group member, discussed the advantages of self-care for her and her clients. The supervisee Betty also realised that her injunction about caring for herself originates from her relationship with her parents. She is taking these themes to her personal therapy.

Vignette 2: "I am like a mountain, with grounded legs": Supervisee rediscovering her strength

In online group supervision with three supervisees, one of the supervisees, Christina, shares her painful countertransference reaction. She feels very uncomfortable with her client, a male around five years older than her. She feels incompetent and insufficient. The client is very passive, and she sometimes wonders why he continues coming. She has a fantasy of him terminating therapy, and then she feels relief. In the previous supervision sessions, the supervision group discussed the client's intrapersonal and relational dynamics and explored the origins of her countertransference from her past. The biggest trigger for her was passiveness, "nothingness" from the client's side, which resembles her father's depressive state. Realising this connection helped her to some extent. The therapy relationship improved and got more vitality. During the last two psychotherapy sessions, she again felt that being with the client was quite unbearable. The client was very passive again, and when she was inquiring about this, his answers felt like they were from another universe, like there was no response from him, even if he answered. In today's supervision session, seeing Christina suffering, the supervisor decides to use the self-compassion processing method (see Chapter 11). Within self-compassion processing, the supervisor also follows the MANER model for self-care.

The supervisor asks the supervisee to imagine the last therapy session with that client and, within it, the most challenging part for her. When she gets the image, the supervisor initiates the first step of MANER; MA: Mindful awareness of body and physiological states.

Supervisor:	*What do you feel in your body now while you are remembering this scene from the last session?*
Supervisee Christina:	*I feel weighed down all over my body and hopelessness.*
Supervisor:	*Christina, if you agree, let's look from a bird's eye perspective at yourself in the last therapy session.*
Supervisee Christina (nodding):	*Ok.*
Supervisor (after a short pause, talking slowly):	*What do you see? What kind of posture do you have? What do you see in your face?*
Supervisee Christina:	*I am bent, my body is bent, and my face is in despair.*

The supervisor initiates step R- regulation and building resources in the following intervention.

Supervisor (gentle, compassionate voice):   Look at yourself with loving eyes.

The supervisor also looks at the supervisee in her imagination and feels a lot of compassion towards her.

Supervisee Christina: I feel a lot of compassion towards myself. I could cry now. I ask myself: why am I doing this work? I don't have to.

The supervisor is present, nodding, and visibly breathing. She is non-verbally supporting and relationally regulating Christina.

Supervisee Christina: I would take me by the hand like this (showing to the group).

The supervisor decides to use the resources of the group. Karin and Irene, the other two group members, also imagine Christina in therapy with that client. The supervisor asks them to share what they see in their imagination.

Supervisee Karin: In my imagination, I am holding you.
Supervisee Irene: I am hugging you.

Her colleagues' supportive and loving words, full of compassion, touch Christina.

Supervisor: Christina, take a breath; what do you feel now?
Supervisee Christina: I feel anger at him.

Christina came into touch with her resources; first self-compassion and then anger. The supervisor now decides to connect this new, resourceful state to her old self-state related to hopelessness. That may promote memory reconsolidation.

Supervisor: If you go back now, in your imagination, to the therapy
                           room, what do you see? What is happening?
Supervisee Christina: I see a similar picture, but I feel different: stronger.
Supervisor: What would you say to Christina?
Supervisee Christina: You don't have to work so hard with him, to suffer so
                           much; let him work harder. (a pause). I don't have to
                           take over so much responsibility, all responsibility;
                           let him take the responsibility, too. And if he feels
                           uncomfortable, so be it.

The supervisor feels empowered and sits up straighter. She uses her experience for the next intervention.

Supervisor: What kind of posture or movement could represent what you have
                just said, your strength?

The supervisee searches for an embodied resource (step R: Regulation and building resources).

Supervisee Christina: I am a mountain; I am like a strong mountain, with
                           grounded legs, strong legs.

The supervisee can use this embodied resource when working with the client.

Supervisor: Yes, feel this ... being a mountain; with strong, grounded legs.

The supervisor is rooting this new, embodied, resourceful experience.

Supervisor (continues):   Feel yourself as a mountain, and think about your
                            next therapy session with that client.

The supervisor invites the supervisee to integrate this new resourceful state with her initial relational schema related to hopelessness and despair.

Supervisee Christina: *Something is pulling me together. I am shrinking; like I am becoming a pile of stones.*

It seems that the supervisee is finding it difficult to stay in touch with this new resource. The supervisor normalises her reaction and explains that her relational matrix with the client is resistant, and she may expect it will not be easy for her during the following psychotherapy sessions. That is why they are preparing her now, at supervision. The supervisor then leads the supervisee to feel like a mountain again. The supervisee connects herself again with the strength and rootedness of the mountain. The supervisor also advises Christina to connect herself with the mountain before the therapy session. The supervisor and supervisees then discuss what may be beneficial for Christina during the therapy session: To be mindful of her feelings and body sensations, and when she starts losing strength, to gently acknowledge that and put herself back in the mountain posture. She should not force herself to become stronger or criticise herself for becoming weaker or desperate because fluctuations in her strength will appear.

At the end of the session, Cristina reflects:

Supervisee Christina: *I am glad we did this. I came into touch with my strengths. I am more prepared now for situations with the client when I start losing myself and my strength. I feel more ready for the therapy sessions.* (pause) *I feel more free now!*

Christina's face looks soft, shining, and rejuvenated.

Vignette 3: Self-care in psychotherapy with the client with borderline features

The supervisee Hana presents the psychotherapy with her client Adriana in the course of triadic supervision. They have been working together for three months of weekly sessions. The supervisee begins by describing how the client has regular fits of jealousy at her partner. She has intense outbursts; she yells and sometimes attacks her husband, throwing and breaking things. The client is traumatised and shows features of borderline personality structure.

Then Hana begins to narrow the question for today's supervision session. She says that the client usually writes to her three times a week. Hana first used to write a short sentence back, but in later sessions, they agreed that the therapist would read the message but won't write back; and they will discuss the subject in the following session.

Supervisee *Hana continues:*	*Yesterday, she wrote me a message that it is difficult for her, and she can't stand it anymore and will leave her husband. I did not respond. I decided I would wait for today's supervision when we can all discuss this together, and you can both help me. It is not difficult for me to work with her; it is pleasant to be with her in the therapy session. She is a great client, opening and developing the capacity for reflection. But how can I help her? That she does not rush into divorce. What can I do? I don't know … I am stuck here.*

While Hana is telling this, the supervisor perceives her as being very calm. The supervisor is also feeling relatively calm, as if feeling nothing special. The supervisor wonders if this calmness is misleading, as it is not congruent with the supervisee's words. She decides to initiate a mindful pause, to provide herself and the supervisees the time and space for awareness of body and emotions. The pause also serves for the first step of MANER, step MA: Mindful awareness of body and physiological states.

Supervisor:	*I would like to ask you, what are you feeling now? Right now, at this moment?* (turns to another supervisee): *Andrew, you also look at yourself, and I will too.*
Supervisee Hana *(inhales and exhales visibly):*	*I feel a slight tension in the area of my stomach; I feel a concern, and maybe a feeling of being powerless.*

The pace is slowing down.

Supervisor:	*Ok. Where in your body do you feel powerlessness?*
Supervisee Hana *(closes her eyes,* *stops for a moment):*	*In my stomach area. Concern and powerlessness; concern in a way that I am worried about powerlessness.*
Supervisor (exhaling *deeply, nodding):*	*What would you say; are you in plus or minus?*

The supervisor asks the supervisee to evaluate her physiological state, referring to the Scale of physiological arousal (G. Žvelc & Žvelc, 2021; see also Chapter 4).

Supervisee Hana:	*Maybe more in minus, more towards hypoarousal.*
Supervisor (nodding, *accepting the* *supervisee's experience):*	*Ok. How much on the scale are you?*

Supervisee Hana:	*−2*
Supervisor:	*According to what signs, would you say that you are in hypo?*
Supervisee Hana (showing a suffering face):	*Because of the fear, this concern, and powerlessness. In this powerlessness, you cannot flee; you cannot fight.*
Supervisor:	*Like some of your functions are switched off.*
Supervisee Hana:	*Yes. Till now, I was not troubled by her. But now, this message that she might leave her husband; this has affected me.* (showing suffering in her face and squeezing her hands in front of her stomach). *It seems to me that her husband is ok, and it would be a pity if she ran away.*

The supervisee Hana is overwhelmed by her concern regarding her client; she is probably merging with her own experience. The supervisor is worried about her welfare. She thinks that Hana might be letting the client come too much into her private space (messages between the sessions, the last message on Sunday evening, intensively worrying about her) and not taking enough care of herself. She wonders if there is some splitting going on, seeing the client as great and vulnerable and not being aware of the demanding and aggressive side of the client, which is crossing her boundaries. The supervisor felt a bit of anger at the client and wondered if the supervisee Hana was disavowing her anger.

Supervisor (to the other supervisee, Andrew):	*What did you notice in your body when we made a mindful pause? If we are not too far from that moment.*
Supervisee Andrew:	*When you asked what we feel in the body, I felt something stopped here, at the area of my chest; something was squeezing me as if I cannot breathe; too much of everything; maybe the client's aggressiveness, destructiveness …. It is demanding work.*

The other supervisee Andrew also feels physiological changes in his body and connects his reaction to the aggressiveness and destructiveness of the client. He also comments that this therapy is demanding. This is significant because it looks as if Hana is avoiding seeing this therapy as demanding and avoiding seeing her client as being aggressive also towards her. The presence of other supervisees is very valuable; they often feel and verbalise what their colleagues are avoiding.

Supervisor:	*Ok. The squeezing, the pressure in the chest. This can also be a sign of immobilisation; like the situation is too bad, it is better not to breathe and better just to hide.*

Supervisor (to Hana):	*How do you explain your body's response, which you have experienced today in supervision?*
Supervisee Hana:	*When I remember yesterday's message from her, which came late, my reaction was, oh, no.* (She puts her head down, indicating a position of powerlessness). *When I saw that she had written to me, I felt it somehow squeezing me. I read it because I promised I would read her messages. Maybe it was not good for me to read it just before going to sleep, and at that moment, I said to myself that I wouldn't read this stuff in the evening; I would wait until the next day because it is essential for me how I sleep. And I was a little angry; there was a mixture of anger at her and at myself for reading it. And in the morning, when I woke up, remembering that we would have supervision today comforted me. At night though, I also had a very uncomfortable dream.*

We see the supervisee is opening up. Before she was unaware of her anger, or maybe she did not allow herself to be angry at the client. Now we see the supervisee's suffering that she was unaware of and unable to reveal to us at the beginning of the session.

Supervisee Hana getting into contact with her anger is a step further. But she is also angry at herself, which shows she may be criticising herself. The supervisor wants to support Hana and lead her towards emotional and physiological regulation. The supervisor also feels the pressure in her own chest and wants to regulate herself. She needs to breathe (step NE: Recognition of needs). By initiating regulation for herself and her supervisees, she is taking step R: Regulation and building resources.

Supervisor:	*Ok. Let us all take a deep breath.*
	(a pause)
Supervisor:	*At the beginning of the session, you, Hana, noticed hypoarousal inside of you, and now you are coming more into touch with your emotions. I think most of what you wanted to put aside was your anger. Metaphorically speaking, maybe you hid it in your stomach. What do you think about what I just said?*

The supervisor connects the supervisee's tension in her stomach with avoiding anger. At the same time, she wants to direct the supervisee's attention to her own anger instead of the client's.

Supervisee Hana:	*Yes, now when you were talking, things come together. I did cut it off* (showing with her hand a cut in front of her stomach).

The supervisor wants to give Hana permission for her anger and show her that it has a significant meaning.

Supervisor:	*The anger you feel has a function. It is significant. It has a meaning. If we look from the evolutionary point of view, it helps us to set boundaries.* (a pause) *How is it for you to read those e-mails? When you see she wrote to you, does it upset you? Do you want to get upset on Sunday evenings?*
Supervisee Hana:	*No. What? No, no, no way* (with a decisive voice, for the first time showing strength in this session).

Letting herself feel the anger and accepting the reality of it, the supervisee can then reflect on it, regulate it, and understand its meaning in relation to the psychotherapy with the client. Anger brings feelings of strength, which can help Hana set boundaries. Clients need compassion and boundaries. And with this kind of attitude, we, as therapists, take care of ourselves too. The therapist has to take care of themselves and the client.

Supervisor (repeats the supervisee's words in a powerful voice):	*No way! Tell us more about that.*
Supervisee Hana:	*This client now writes to me three times every week. In the beginning, I wrote back to say that I had heard her; later, I thought I couldn't ignore her, so I said I would read her messages, but not answer them. I don't know what I was thinking; I wanted to calm her down.*
Supervisor:	*You wanted to be a good mother.*
Supervisee Hana:	*A good mother, yes. And now I am angry, mostly at myself.*
Supervisor:	*I would like to normalise that this is a typical countertransference with clients with borderline features. They are pulling us in … and also touching our wounds … I know that you know that …*
Supervisee Hana:	*Yes, when you are pulled in, things are different; you don't see clearly anymore.*
Supervisor:	*We are pulled into the state where we want to be good, provide the clients with what they missed, and give them the best.* (pause) *In the therapeutic session, we are there for them. But if we want to give more than the professional relationship can offer, this is not professional, it can be counterproductive, and complicates the therapy. The anger you feel, if you don't use it for self-criticism, can be constructive and help you to decide: I will do this differently, I will set boundaries. I deserve my space; I deserve a good night's sleep.*

Supervisee Hana: *I feel decisiveness in myself. As you said, the anger at this moment is working for me; helping me to set boundaries. And also, in my body, the energy has shifted to here* (indicating her chest), *and I feel decisiveness and strength. Now I am at zero* (referring to the Scale of physiological arousal, where zero is the balanced, optimal arousal).

Supervision is now successfully fulfilling step R: Regulation and building resources.

Supervisor: *Ok. So, what can you do differently?*

The supervisee Hana, at this point, becomes physiologically regulated and enters the window of tolerance; she comes into touch with her strength as a resource for her needs. Now it is time to return to Hana's initial question regarding how to react to Adriana's messages. Now it's time to move from the supervisee's regulated emotions and physiology to a more cognitive decision-making part. Hana shares some ideas, and then with Andrew and the supervisor, they discuss possible ways of setting boundaries for the client. They also talk about how to support the client. They discuss and find new ways to help the client regulate herself during therapy and outside of it. The more the client can come to regulate herself, the fewer messages she would need to send and make less impulsive decisions. At the end of the supervision session, they come back to supervisee Hana's vulnerable part and her suffering, which was revealed in the course of the session. Hana's anger during the supervision session transformed into strength and compassion for herself and the client. The supervisor encourages Hana that after the supervision session, she writes down all the supporting words she would like to say to herself; and read these words before the therapy with Adriana. In supervision, we want the supervisees to recognise their own suffering connected to working with clients; and provide care, kindness, and support to themselves. They may also need to bring their personal issues triggered by the work to their personal psychotherapy, as Hana did.

A frequent psychotherapist's countertransference when working with clients with borderline features is wanting to give them the love, attention, and protection they missed so much in their childhood. They adjust to their clients' wishes too much, let them cross their professional boundaries, and then they become exhausted and drained because there is never enough. And finally, therapists get angry at their clients for what they are doing to them. In this way, therapists are caught in the relational enactment, pulled to give those clients more than they give the "average" client. Also, our supervisee Hana was stuck in her helping role as a preoccupied "mother". The client had intense separation anxiety, and the supervisee was somehow caught in the enactment, wanting to heal this deep client's wound. The wound of the client resonates with the supervisee's wound. The supervisee had difficulties in recognising that the client is very demanding and that she is giving too much, more than her professional role asks her to. What the client wants is not necessarily the same as what the client needs.

If the supervisee Hana sets the boundaries respectfully, she also models the client on how to set boundaries in an appropriate way instead of throwing things around and attacking her husband. In some way, the client may unconsciously cross the therapist's boundaries to see how the therapist will cope with that. Unconsciously, she may want to see and learn how to set boundaries. Her boundaries were severely crossed in her life, and by crossing the therapist's boundaries, she is unconsciously revealing her story to the therapist. In every enactment, there is also hope for reparation – in this client's case, a need to see how someone can, in a respectful way, set an appropriate boundary.

When the therapist fails to recognise this and stays merged with the client's dysregulated physiology, they are getting drawn into a state of emotional stress and exhaustion. Here, the supervision third eye is needed. Supervision needs to reveal this relational enactment and help the therapist reestablish a decentred perspective, as seen in this last vignette.

During the presented supervision session, Hana's experience of excessive concern and powerlessness transformed first into feelings of anger and then into strength and self-compassion. During the supervision session, she also internalised the skill of moment-to-moment mindful awareness of body sensations and needs and the significance of physiological regulation. From this, she can lead the subsequent therapies with compassionate care for herself and the client.

Appendix

Online supplements

Online resources for the readers of *Mindfulness and Compassion in Integrative Supervision* are available at: www.mcip.eu

Supplements include scales for researchers and clinicians, case presentation resources, and other related materials.

References

Allen, G. J., Szollos, S. J., & Williams, B. E. (1986). Doctoral students' comparative evaluations of best and worst psychotherapy supervision. *Professional Psychology: Research and Practice, 17*(2), 91–99. https://doi.org/10.1037//0735-7028.17.2.91

Alonso, A., & Rutan, J. S. (1988). Shame and guilt in psychotherapy supervision. *Psychotherapy, 25*(4), 576–581. https://doi.org/10.1037/h0085384

Angus, L., & Kagan, F. (2007). Empathic relational bonds and personal agency in psychotherapy: Implications for psychotherapy supervision, practice, and research. *Psychotherapy, 44*(4), 371–377. https://doi.org/10.1037/0033-3204.44.4.371

Arch, J. J., Brown, K. W., Dean, D. J., Landy, L. N., Brown, K. D., & Laudenslager, M. L. (2014). Self-compassion training modulates alpha-amylase, heart rate variability, and subjective responses to social evaluative threat in women. *Psychoneuroendocrinology, 42,* 49–58. https://doi.org/10.1016/j.psyneuen.2013.12.018

Atkinson, D. M., Rodman, J. L., Thuras, P. D., Shiroma, P. R., & Lim, K. O. (2017). Examining burnout, depression, and self-compassion in veterans affairs mental health staff. *Journal of Alternative and Complementary Medicine, 23*(7), 551–557. https://doi.org/10.1089/acm.2017.0087

Banker, J. E., & Goldenson, D. (2021). Mindfulness practices in supervision: Training counselors' experiences. *Family Journal, 29*(1), 17–23. https://doi.org/10.1177/10664 80720954204

Bar-Kalifa, E., Prinz, J. N., Atzil-Slonim, D., Rubel, J. A., Lutz, W., & Rafaeli, E. (2019). Physiological synchrony and therapeutic alliance in an imagery-based treatment. *Journal of Counseling Psychology, 66*(4), 508–517. https://doi.org/10.1037/cou0000358

Barlow, M. R., Goldsmith, R. E., & Gerhart, J. (2017). Trauma appraisals, emotion regulation difficulties, and self-compassion predict posttraumatic stress symptoms following childhood abuse. *Child Abuse & Neglect, 65,* 37–47. https://doi.org/10.1016/j.chiabu.2017.01.006

Bateman, A., & Fonagy, P. (2016). *Mentalization-based treatment for personality disorders: A practical guide.* Oxford University Press.

Bates, G. W., Elphinstone, B., & Whitehead, R. (2021). Self-compassion and emotional regulation as predictors of social anxiety. *Psychology and Psychotherapy: Theory, Research and Practice, 94,* 426–442. https://doi.org/10.1111/papt.12318

Beaumont, E., Rayner, G., Durkin, M., & Bowling, G. (2017). The effects of compassionate mind training on student psychotherapists. *Journal of Mental Health*

Training, Education and Practice, 12(5), 300–312. https://doi.org/10.1108/JMHTEP-06-2016-0030

Bell, T., Dixon, A., & Kolts, R. (2017). Developing a compassionate internal supervisor: Compassion-focused therapy for trainee therapists. *Clinical Psychology and Psychotherapy, 24*(3), 632–648. https://doi.org/10.1002/cpp.2031

Bennett, C. S. (2008). The interface of attachment, transference, and countertransference: Implications for the clinical supervisory relationship. *Smith College Studies in Social Work, 78*(2–3), 301–320. https://doi.org/10.1080/00377310802114635

Bordin, E. S. (1983). A working alliance based model of supervision. *The Counseling Psychologist, 11*(1), 35–42.

Brach, T. (2012). Mindful presence: A foundation for compassion and wisdom. In C. K. Germer & R. D. Siegel (Eds.), *Wisdom and compassion in psychotherapy: Deepening mindfulness in clinical practice* (pp. 35–47). The Guilford Press.

Brach, T. (2020). *Radical compassion: Learning to love yourself and your world with the practice of RAIN.* Rider.

Breines, J. G., McInnis, C. M., Kuras, Y. I., Thoma, M. V., Gianferante, D., Hanlin, L., Chen, X., & Rohleder, N. (2015). Self-compassionate young adults show lower salivary alpha-amylase responses to repeated psychosocial stress. *Self and Identity, 14*(4), 390–402. https://doi.org/10.1080/15298868.2015.1005659

Buber, M. (1999). *Princip dialoga [The dialogic principle] (J. Zupet, Trans.).* Društvo izdajateljev časnika 2000.

Buchanan, T. W., Bagley, S. L., Stansfield, R. B., & Preston, S. D. (2012). The empathic, physiological resonance of stress. *Social Neuroscience, 7*(2), 191–201. https://doi.org/10.1080/17470919.2011.588723

Carter, J. W., Enyedy, K. C., Goodyear, R. K., Arcinue, F., & Puri, N. N. (2009). Concept mapping of the events supervisees find helpful in group supervision. *Training and Education in Professional Psychology, 3*(1), 1–9. https://doi.org/10.1037/a0013656

Casement, P. (1985). *On learning from the patient.* Tavistock.

Casement, P. (1990). *Further learning from the patient: The analytic space and process.* Brunner-Routledge.

Casement, P. (2002). *Learning from our mistakes: Beyond dogma in psychoanalysis and psychotherapy.* Guilford Press.

Cavicchioli, M., Movalli, M., & Maffei, C. (2018). The clinical efficacy of mindfulness-based treatments for alcohol and drugs use disorders: A meta-analytic review of randomized and nonrandomized controlled trials. *European Addiction Research, 24*(3), 137–162. https://doi.org/10.1159/000490762

Chalikkandy, S., Alhifzi, R. S. A., Asiri, M. A. Y., Alshahrani, R. S. A., Saeed, W. N. A., & Alamri, S. G. (2022). Burnout and its relation to emotion dysregulation and social cognition among female interns and undergraduate dental students at King Khalid University. *Applied Sciences, 12*(3), 1–10. https://doi.org/10.3390/app12031588

Champe, J., Okech, J. E. A., & Rubel, D. J. (2013). Emotion regulation: Processes, strategies, and applications to group work training and supervision. *Journal for Specialists in Group Work, 38*(4), 349–368. https://doi.org/10.1080/01933922.2013.834403

Coaston, S. C. (2017). Self-care through self-compassion: A balm for burnout. *The Professional Counselor, 7*(3), 285–297. https://doi.org/10.15241/scc.7.3.285

Coaston, S. C. (2019). Cultivating self-compassion within the supervision relationship. *Clinical Supervisor*, *38*(1), 79–96. https://doi.org/10.1080/07325223.2018.1525596

Crunk, A. E., & Barden, S. M. (2017). The common factors discrimination model: An integrated approach to counselor supervision. *The Professional Counselor*, *7*(1), 62–75. https://doi.org/10.15241/aec.7.1.62

Dana, D. (2018). *The polyvagal theory in therapy: Engaging the rhythm of regulation*. W.W. Norton & Company.

Davidson, C. (2011). The relation between supervisor self-disclosure and the working alliance among social work students in field placement. *Journal of Teaching in Social Work*, *31*(3), 265–277. https://doi.org/10.1080/08841233.2011.580248

Deikman, A. J. (1982). *The observing self: Mysticism and psychotherapy*. Beacon Press.

Desmond, T. (2016). *Self-compassion in psychotherapy: Mindfulness-based practices for healing and transformation*. W.W. Norton & Company.

di Pellegrino, G., Fadiga, L., Fogassi, L., Gallese, V., & Rizzolatti, G. (1992). Understanding motor events: A neurophysiological study. *Experimental Brain Research*, *91*(1), 176–180. https://doi.org/10.1007/BF00230027

Dickson, J. M., Moberly, N. J., Marshall, Y., & Reilly, J. (2011). Attachment style and its relationship to working alliance in the supervision of British clinical psychology trainees. *Clinical Psychology and Psychotherapy*, *18*(4), 322–330. https://doi.org/10.1002/cpp.715

Diedrich, A., Burger, J., Kirchner, M., & Berking, M. (2016). Adaptive emotion regulation mediates the relationship between self-compassion and depression in individuals with unipolar depression. *Psychology & Psychotherapy: Theory, Research, and Practice*, *90*(3), 247–263. https://doi.org/10.1111/papt.12107

Dreisoerner, A., Junker, N. M., Schlotz, W., Heimrich, J., Bloemeke, S., Ditzen, B., & van Dick, R. (2021). Self-soothing touch and being hugged reduce cortisol responses to stress: A randomized controlled trial on stress, physical touch, and social identity. *Comprehensive Psychoneuroendocrinology*, *8*. https://doi.org/10.1016/j.cpnec.2021.100091

Ecker, B. (2015). Memory reconsolidation understood and misunderstood. *International Journal of Neuropsychotherapy*, *3*, 2–46. https://doi.org/10.12744/ijnpt.2015.0002-0046

Ecker, B. (2018). Clinical translation of memory reconsolidation research: Therapeutic methodology for transformational change by erasing implicit emotional learnings driving symptom production. *International Journal of Neuropsychotherapy*, *6*(1), 1–92. https://doi.org/10.12744/ijnpt.2018.0001-0092

Ecker, B., Robin, T., & Hulley, L. (2012). *Unlocking the emotional brain: Eliminating symptoms at their roots using memory reconsolidation*. Routledge.

Ecker, B., & Vaz, A. (2019, June 6–8). Beyond common and specific factors: Memory reconsolidation as a transtheoretical mechanism of change and unifying framework in psychotherapy [Conference session]. SEPI XXXV Annual Meeting, Lisbon, Portugal.

Elliott, R. (2010). Psychotherapy change process research: Realizing the promise. *Psychotherapy Research*, *20*(2), 123–135. https://doi.org/10.1080/10503300903470743

Elliott, R., Slatick, E., & Urman, M. (2001). Qualitative change process research on psychotherapy: Alternative strategies. In J. Frommer & D. L. Rennie (Eds.), *Qualitative psychotherapy research: Methods and methodology* (pp. 69–111). Pabst Science Publishers.

Ellis, M. V. (2001). Harmful supervision, a cause for alarm: Comment on Gray et al. (2001) and Nelson and Friedlander (2001). *Journal of Counseling Psychology, 48*(4), 401–406.

Ellis, M. V., Berger, L., Hanus, A. E., Ayala, E. E., Swords, B. A., & Siembor, M. (2014). Inadequate and harmful clinical supervision: Testing a revised framework and assessing occurrence. *The Counseling Psychologist, 42*(4), 434–472. https://doi.org/10.1177/0011000013508656

Engler, J., & Fulton, P. R. (2012). Self and no-self in psychotherapy. In C. K. Germer & R. D. Siegel (Eds.), *Wisdom and compassion in psychotherapy: Deepening mindfulness in clinical practice* (pp. 176–189). The Guilford Press.

Eriksson, T., Germundsjö, L., Åström, E., & Rönnlund, M. (2018). Mindful self-compassion training reduces stress and burnout symptoms among practicing psychologists: A randomized controlled trial of a brief web-based intervention. *Frontiers in Psychology, 9*, 1–10. https://doi.org/10.3389/fpsyg.2018.02340

Erskine, R. G. (1982). Supervision of psychotherapy: Models for professional development. *Transactional Analysis Journal, 12*(4), 314–321.

Erskine, R. G. (1993). Inquiry, attunement, and involvement in the psychotherapy of dissociation. *Transactional Analysis Journal, 23*(4), 184–190. https://doi.org/10.1177/036215379302300402

Erskine, R. G. (2015). *Relational patterns, therapeutic presence: Concepts and practice of integrative psychotherapy.* Karnac Books.

Erskine, R. G. (2020). Compassion, hope, and forgiveness in the therapeutic dialogue. *International Journal of Integrative Psychotherapy, 11*(1), 1–13.

Erskine, R. G., & Moursund, J. P. (2011). *Integrative psychotherapy in action* (2nd ed.). Karnac Books.

Erskine, R. G., & Moursund, J. P. (2022). *The art and science of relationship: The practice of integrative psychotherapy* (2nd ed.). Phoenix Publishing House.

Erskine, R. G., Moursund, J. P., & Trautmann, R. L. (1999). *Beyond empathy: A therapy of contact-in-relationship.* Brunner/Mazel.

Erskine, R. G., Moursund, J. P., & Trautmann R. L. (2023). *Beyond empathy: A therapy of contact-in-relationship* (Classic ed.). Routledge.

Erskine, R. G., & Trautmann, R. L. (1996). Methods of an integrative psychotherapy. *Transactional Analysis Journal, 26*(4), 316–328. https://doi.org/10.1177/036215379602600410

Erskine, R. G., & Trautmann, R. L. (1997). The process of integrative psychotherapy. In *Theories and methods of an integrative transactional analysis: A volume of selected articles* (pp. 79–95). TA Press. (Original work published 1993).

Eubanks, C. F., Muran, J. C., & Safran, J. D. (2018). Alliance rupture repair: A meta-analysis. *Psychotherapy, 55*(4), 508–519. https://doi.org/10.1037/pst0000185

Evans, A. J. (2018). *Perspectives of mindfulness-based supervision: A grounded theory study.* University of Exeter.

Farb, N. A. S., Anderson, A. K., & Segal, Z. V. (2012). The mindful brain and emotion regulation in mood disorders. *Canadian Journal of Psychiatry, 57*(2), 70–77. https://doi.org/10.1177/070674371205700203

Farb, N. A. S., Segal, Z. V., Mayberg, H., Bean, J., Mckeon, D., Fatima, Z., & Anderson, A. K. (2007). Attending to the present: Mindfulness meditation reveals distinct neural modes of self-reference. *Social Cognitive and Affective Neuroscience, 2*(4), 313–322. https://doi.org/10.1093/scan/nsm030

Farb, N., Daubenmier, J., Price, C. J., Gard, T., Kerr, C., Dunn, B. D., Klein, A. C., Paulus, M. P., & Mehling, W. E. (2015). Interoception, contemplative practice, and health. *Frontiers in Psychology, 6*, 1–26. https://doi.org/10.3389/fpsyg.2015.00763

Felton, T. M., Coates, L., & Christopher, J. C. (2015). Impact of mindfulness training on counseling students' perceptions of stress. *Mindfulness, 6*(2), 159–169. https://doi.org/10.1007/s12671-013-0240-8

Ferrari, M., Hunt, C., Harrysunker, A., Abbott, M. J., Beath, A. P., & Einstein, D. A. (2019). Self-compassion interventions and psychosocial outcomes: A meta-analysis of RCTs. *Mindfulness, 10*, 1455–1473. https://doi.org/10.1007/s12671-019-01134-6

Ferrari, P. F., & Gallese, V. (2007). Mirror neurons and intersubjectivity. In S. Bråten (Ed.), *On being moved from mirror neurons to empathy* (Vol. 1, pp. 73–88). John Benjamins Publishing Company. https://doi.org/10.1075/aicr.68.08fer

Finlay-Jones, A. L. (2017). The relevance of self-compassion as an intervention target in mood and anxiety disorders: A narrative review based on an emotion regulation framework. *Clinical Psychologist, 21*(2), 90–103. https://doi.org/10.1111/cp.12131

Fletcher, L., Pond, R., Gardiner, B., Fletcher, L., Pond, R., Gardiner, B., Fletcher, L., Pond, R., & Gardiner, B. (2022). Student counsellor experiences of mindfulness-based intervention training: A systematic review of the qualitative literature. *Psychotherapy Research, 32*(3), 306–328. https://doi.org/10.1080/10503307.2021.1946615

Fonagy, P., Gergely, G., Jurist, E. L., & Target, M. (2004). *Affect regulation, mentalization, and the development of the self.* Karnac.

Fosha, D. (2000a). Meta-therapeutic processes and the affects of transformation: Affirmation and the healing affects. *Journal of Psychotherapy Integration, 10*(1), 71–97. https://doi.org/10.1023/A:1009422511959

Fosha, D. (2000b). *The transforming power of affect: A model for accelerated change.* Basic Books.

Fosha, D., & Conceição, N. (2019). How to be a transformational therapist and integrate transformational work into your clinical practice: Insights from the clinical practice of and research into AEDP [Conference session]. *SEPI 35th Annual Meeting*, Lisbon, Portugal, June 6–8.

Fosha, D., Thoma, N., & Yeung, D. (2019). Transforming emotional suffering into flourishing: Metatherapeutic processing of positive affect as a trans-theoretical vehicle for change. *Counselling Psychology Quarterly, 32*(3–4), 563–593. https://doi.org/10.1080/09515070.2019.1642852

Frawley-O'Dea, M. G., & Sarnat, J. E. (2001). *The supervisory relationship: A contemporary psychodynamic approach.* Guilford Press.

Garrote-Caparrós, E., Bellosta-Batalla, M., & Moya-Albiol, L. (2022). Effectiveness of mindfulness-based interventions on psychotherapy processes: A systematic review. *Clinical Psychology & Psychotherapy, 29*, 783–798. https://doi.org/10.1002/cpp.2676

Geller, J. D., Farber, B. A., & Schaffer, C. E. (2010). Representations of the supervisory dialogue and the development of psychotherapists. *Psychotherapy, 47*(2), 211–220. https://doi.org/10.1037/a0019785

Geller, S. M. (2018). Therapeutic presence and polyvagal theory. Principles and practices for cultivating effective therapeutic relationships. In S. W. Porges & D. Dana (Eds.), *Clinical applications of the polyvagal theory. The emergence of polyvagal-informed therapies* (pp. 106–126). W.W. Norton & Company.

Geller, S. M., & Greenberg, L. S. (2012). *Therapeutic presence. A mindful approach to effective therapy*. American Psychological Association.

Geller, S. M., & Porges, S. W. (2014). Therapeutic presence: Neurophysiological mechanisms mediating feeling safe in therapeutic relationships. *Journal of Psychotherapy Integration, 24*, 178–192. https://doi.org/10.1037/a0037511

Germer, C. K. (2012). Cultivating compassion in psychotherapy. In C. K. Germer & R. D. Siegel (Eds.), *Wisdom and compassion in psychotherapy: Deepening mindfulness in clinical practice* (pp. 93–110). Guilford Press.

Germer, C., & Neff, K. (2013). The mindful self-compassion training program. In T. Singer & M. Bolz (Eds.), *Compassion: Bridging practice and science* (pp. 364–396). Max-Planck Institute.

Gilbert, M. C., & Evans, K. (2000). *Psychotherapy supervision: An integrative relational approach to psychotherapy supervision*. Open University Press.

Gilbert, P. (2009). *The compassionate mind: A new approach to life's challenges*. New Harbinger Publications, Inc.

Gilbert, P. (2010). *Compassion focused therapy: Distinctive features*. Routledge.

Gilbert, P., & Procter, S. (2006). Compassionate mind training for people with high shame and self-criticism: Overview and pilot study of a group therapy approach. *Clinical Psychology and Psychotherapy, 13*(6), 353–379. https://doi.org/10.1002/cpp.507

Goldberg, S. B., Tucker, R. P., Greene, P. A., Davidson, R. J., Wampold, B. E., Kearney, D. J., & Simpson, T. L. (2018). Mindfulness-based interventions for psychiatric disorders: A systematic review and meta-analysis. *Clinical Psychology Review, 59*, 52–60. https://doi.org/10.1016/j.cpr.2017.10.011

Goldin, P. R., & Gross, J. J. (2010). Effects of mindfulness-based stress reduction (MBSR) on emotion regulation in social anxiety disorder. *Emotion, 10*(1), 83–91. https://doi.org/10.1037/a0018441

Graff, G. (2008). Shame in supervision. *Issues in Psychoanalytic Psychology, 30*(1), 79–94.

Grant, J., Schofield, M. M., & Crawford, S. (2012). Managing difficulties in supervision: Supervisors' perspectives. *Journal of Counseling Psychology, 59*(4), 528–541. https://doi.org/10.1037/a0030000

Gray, L. A., Ladany, N., Walker, J. A., & Ancis, J. R. (2001). Psychotherapy trainees' experience of counterproductive events in supervision. *Journal of Counseling Psychology, 48*(4), 371–383. https://doi.org/10.1037/0022-0167.48.4.371

Greenberg, L. S. (1986). Change process research. *Journal of Consulting and Clinical Psychology, 54*(1), 4–9.

Gross, J. J. (2001). Emotion regulation in adulthood: Timing is everything. *Current Directions in Psychological Science, 10*(6), 214–219. https://doi.org/10.1111/1467-8721.00152

Guistolise, P. G. (1996). Failures in the therapeutic relationship: Inevitable and necessary? *Transactional Analysis Journal, 26*(4), 284–288. https://doi.org/10.1177/036215379602600403

Haberlin, S. (2020). Mindfulness-based supervision: Awakening to new possibilities. *Journal of Educational Supervision, 3*(3), 75–89. https://doi.org/10.31045/jes.3.3.6

Hahn, W. K. (2001). The experience of shame in psychotherapy supervision. *Psychotherapy, 38*(3), 272–282.

Hatfield, E., Bensman, L., Thornton, P. D., & Rapson, R. L. (2014). New perspectives on emotional contagion: A review of classic and recent research on facial mimicry and contagion. *Interpersona: An International Journal on Personal Relationships*, *8*(2), 159–179. https://doi.org/10.5964/ijpr.v8i2.162

Hawkins, P., & Shohet, R. (2012). *Supervision in the helping professions*. Open University Press.

Hayes, A. M., & Feldman, G. (2004). Clarifying the construct of mindfulness in the context of emotion regulation and the process of change in therapy. *Clinical Psychology: Science and Practice*, *11*(3), 255–262. https://doi.org/10.1093/clipsy/bph080

Hayes, S. C. (1984). Making sense of spirituality. *Behaviorism*, *12*, 99–110. https://contextualscience.org/files/Hayes1984.pdf

Hayes, S. C., & Hofmann, S. G. (2018). Introduction. In S. C. Hayes & S. G. Hofmann (Eds.), *Process-based CBT: The science and core clinical competencies of cognitive behavioral therapy* (pp. 1–7). Context Press: An Imprint of New Harbinger Publications, Inc.

Hayes, S. C., & Spencer, S. (2005). *Get out of your mind & into your life: The new acceptance and commitment therapy*. New Harbinger Publications, Inc.

Hayes, S. C., Strosahl, K. D., & Wilson, K. G. (1999). *Acceptance and commitment therapy: An experiential approach to behavior change*. The Guilford Press.

Hayes, S. C., Strosahl, K. D., & Wilson, K. G. (2012). *Acceptance and commitment therapy: The process and practice of mindful change* (2nd ed.). The Guilford Press.

Helm, J. L., Sbarra, D. A., & Ferrer, E. (2014). Coregulation of respiratory sinus arrhythmia in adult romantic partners. *Emotion*, *14*(3), 522–531. https://doi.org/10.1037/a0035960

Henderson, C. E., Cawyer, C. S., & Watkins, C. E. (1999). A comparison of student and supervisor perceptions of effective practicum supervision. *Clinical Supervisor*, *18*(1), 47–74. https://doi.org/10.1300/J001v18n01_04

Hiebler-Ragger, M., Nausner, L., Blaha, A., Grimmer, K., Korlath, S., Mernyi, M., & Unterrainer, H. F. (2021). The supervisory relationship from an attachment perspective: Connections to burnout and sense of coherence in health professionals. *Clinical Psychology and Psychotherapy*, *28*(1), 124–136. https://doi.org/10.1002/cpp.2494

Hill, D. (2015). *Affect regulation theory: A clinical model*. W.W. Norton & Company.

Hofmann, S. G., & Hayes, S. C. (2019). The future of intervention science: Process-based therapy. *Clinical Psychological Science*, *7*(1), 37–50. https://doi.org/10.1177/2167702618772296

Hofmeyer, A., Kennedy, K., & Taylor, R. (2020). Contesting the term 'compassion fatigue': Integrating findings from social neuroscience and self-care research. *Collegian*, *27*(2), 232–237. https://doi.org/10.1016/j.colegn.2019.07.001

Holloway, E. L. (1987). Developmental models of supervision: Is it development? *Professional Psychology: Research and Practice*, *18*(3), 209–216. https://doi.org/10.1037/0735-7028.18.3.209

Hölzel, B. K., Lazar, S. W., Gard, T., Schuman-Olivier, Vago, D. R., & Ott, U. (2011). How does mindfulness meditation work. *Perspectives on Psychological Science*, *6*(6), 537–559. https://doi.org/10.1177/1745691611419671

Hsu, S., & Tsai, S. (2006). Dropout from supervision: An intensive analysis of one supervisory dyad. *Bulletin of Educational Psychology*, *38*(2), 213–225.

Hutt, C. H., Scott, J., & King, M. (1983). A phenomenological study of supervisees' positive and negative experiences in supervision. *Psychotherapy: Theory, Research and Practice, 20*, 118–123.

Inwood, E., & Ferrari, M. (2018). Mechanisms of change in the relationship between self-compassion, emotion regulation, and mental health: A systematic review. *Health and Well-Being, 10*(2), 215–235. https://doi.org/10.1111/aphw.12127

Iraurgi, I., Gómez-Marroquín, I., Erskine, R., Mauriz, A., Martínez-Rodríguez, S., Gorbeña, S., & Žvelc, G. (2022). Adaptation to Spanish of the "relational needs satisfaction scale": Translation and psychometric testing. *Frontiers in Psychology, 13*, 1–12. https://doi.org/10.3389/fpsyg.2022.992205

Jackson-Koku, G., & Grime, P. (2019). Emotion regulation and burnout in doctors: A systematic review. *Occupational Medicine, 69*(1), 9–21. https://doi.org/10.1093/occmed/kqz004

Jacobsen, C. H., & Tanggaard, L. (2009). Beginning therapists' experiences of what constitutes good and bad psychotherapy supervision with a special focus on individual differences. *Nordic Psychology, 61*(4), 59–84. https://doi.org/10.1027/1901-2276.61.4.59

Kabat-Zinn, J. (1990). *Full catastrophe living: How to cope with stress, pain and illness using mindfulness meditation.* Piatkos.

Kabat-Zinn, J. (1994). *Wherever you go, there you are: Mindfulness meditation in everyday life.* Hyperion.

Karvonen, A., Kykyri, V. L., Kaartinen, J., Penttonen, M., & Seikkula, J. (2016). Sympathetic nervous system synchrony in couple therapy. *Journal of Marital and Family Therapy, 42*(3), 383–395. https://doi.org/10.1111/jmft.12152

Kastelic, K., Kralj, M., & Črnigoj, P. (2022). *Izgorelost, sočutje do sebe in težave v uravnavanju čustev pri psihoterapevtih [Burnout, self-compassion and affect regulation problems among psychotherapists]* (Research report). Institute IPSA.

Keil, M. S. (2016). *Mindfulness in clinical supervision: Impacts on the working alliance and supervisees' perceptions of self-efficacy.* ProQuest Dissertations Publishing [Doctoral dissertation]. Azusa Pacific University.

Kleinbub, J. R. (2017). State of the art of interpersonal physiology in psychotherapy: A systematic review. *Frontiers in Psychology, 8.* https://doi.org/10.3389/fpsyg.2017.02053

Kleinbub, J. R., Talia, A., & Palmieri, A. (2020). Physiological synchronization in the clinical process: A research primer. *Journal of Counseling Psychology, 67*(4), 420–437. https://doi.org/10.1037/cou0000383

Klimecki, O., & Singer, T. (2012). Empathic distress fatigue rather than compassion fatigue? Integrating findings from empathy research in psychology and social neuroscience. In B. Oakley, A. Knafo, G. Madhavan, & D. S. Wilson (Eds.), *Pathological altruism* (pp. 368–383). Oxford University Press. https://doi.org/10.1093/acprof

Klimecki, O. M., Leiberg, S., Ricard, M., & Singer, T. (2013). Differential pattern of functional brain plasticity after compassion and empathy training. *Social Cognitive and Affective Neuroscience, 9*(6), 873–879. https://doi.org/10.1093/scan/nst060

Knox, S., Burkard, A. W., Edwards, L. M., Smith, J. J., & Schlosser, L. Z. (2008). Supervisors' reports of the effects of supervisor self-disclosure on supervisees. *Psychotherapy Research, 18*, 543–559. https://doi.org/10.1080/10503300801982781

Knox, S., Edwards, L. M., Hess, S. A., & Hill, C. E. (2011). Supervisor self-disclosure: Supervisees' experiences and perspectives. *Psychotherapy*, *48*(4), 336–341. https://doi.org/10.1037/a0022067

Kotera, Y., Maxwell-Jones, R., Edwards, A. M., & Knutton, N. (2021). Burnout in professional psychotherapists: Relationships with self-compassion, work–life balance, and telepressure. *International Journal of Environmental Research and Public Health*, *18*(10). https://doi.org/10.3390/ijerph18105308

Ladany, N., & Lehrman-Waterman, D. E. (1999). The content and frequency of supervisor self-disclosures and their relationship to supervisor style and the supervisory working alliance. *Counselor Education & Supervision*, *38*(3), 143–160.

Ladany, N., Ellis, M. V., & Friedlander, M. L. (1999). The supervisory working alliance, trainee self-efficacy, and satisfaction. *Journal of Counseling & Development*, *77*(4), 447–455. https://doi.org/10.1002/j.1556-6676.1999.tb02472.x

Ladany, N., Friedlander, M. L., & Nelson, M. L. (2005). *Critical events in psychotherapy supervision: An interpersonal approach*. American Psychological Association.

Ladany, N., Hill, C. E., Corbett, M. M., & Nutt, E. A. (1996). Nature, extent, and importance of what psychotherapy trainees do not disclose to their supervisors. *Journal of Counseling Psychology*, *43*(1), 10–24. https://doi.org/10.1037/0022-0167.43.1.10

Ladany, N., Walker, J. A., & Melincoff, D. S. (2001). Supervisory style: Its relation to the supervisory working alliance and supervisor self-disclosure. *Counselor Education & Supervision*, *40*, 263–275.

Lampropoulos, G. K. (2003). A common factors view of counseling supervision process. *Clinical Supervisor*, *21*(1), 77–95. https://doi.org/10.1300/J001v21n01_06

Lane, R. D., Lee, R., Nadel, L., & Greenberg, L. (2015). Memory reconsolidation, emotional arousal, and the process of change in psychotherapy: New insights from brain science. *Behavioral and Brain Sciences*, *38*, 1–64. https://doi.org/10.1017/S0140525X14000041

Langs, R. (1994). *Doing supervision and being supervised*. Karnac.

Leary, M. R., Tate, E. B., Adams, C. E., Allen, A. B., & Hancock, J. (2007). Self-compassion and reactions to unpleasant self-relevant events: The implications of treating oneself kindly. *Journal of Personality and Social Psychology*, *92*(5), 887–904. https://doi.org/10.1037/0022-3514.92.5.887

Lee, J., Lim, N., Yang, E., & Lee, S. M. (2011). Antecedents and consequences of three dimensions of burnout in psychotherapists: A meta-analysis. *Professional Psychology: Research and Practice*, *42*(3), 252–258. https://doi.org/10.1037/a0023319

Levine, P. A. (1997). *Waking the tiger: Healing trauma*. North Atlantic Books.

Levine, P. A. (2018). Polyvagal theory and trauma. In S. W. Porges & D. Dana (Eds.), *Clinical applications of the Polyvagal theory. The emergence of polyvagal-infromed therapies* (pp. 3–26). W.W. Norton & Company.

Ley, R. (1994). Breathing and the psychology of emotion, cognition, and behavior. In B. H. Timmons & R. Ley (Eds.), *Behavioral and psychological approaches to breathing disorders* (pp. 81–95). Plenum Press. https://doi.org/10.1007/978-1-4757-9383-3_6

Lindsay, E. K., & Creswell, J. D. (2019). Mindfulness, acceptance, and emotion regulation: Perspectives from monitor and acceptance theory (MAT). *Current Opinion in Psychology*, *28*, 120–125. https://doi.org/10.1016/j.copsyc.2018.12.004

Luoma, J. B., Hayes, S. C., & Walser, R. D. (2007). *Learning ACT: An acceptance & commitment therapy skills-training manual for therapists.* New Harbinger Publications, Inc.

Lyons-Ruth, K., Bruschweiler-Stern, N., Harrison, A. M., Morgan, A. C., Nahum, J. P., Sander, L., Stern, D. N., & Tronick, E. Z. (1998). Implicit relational knowing: Its role in development and psychoanalytic treatment. *Infant Mental Health Journal, 19*(3), 282–289.

MacBeth, A., & Gumley, A. (2012). Exploring compassion: A meta-analysis of the association between self-compassion and psychopathology. *Clinical Psychology Review, 32*(6), 545–552. https://doi.org/10.1016/j.cpr.2012.06.003

Mantelou, A., & Karakasidou, E. (2019). The role of compassion for self and others, compassion fatigue and subjective happiness on levels of well-being of mental health professionals. *Psychology, 10*, 285–304. https://doi.org/10.4236/psych.2019.103021

Marci, C. D., Ham, J., Moran, E., & Orr, S. P. (2007). Physiologic correlates of perceived therapist empathy and social-emotional process during psychotherapy. *Journal of Nervous and Mental Disease, 195*(2), 103–111. https://doi.org/10.1097/01.nmd.0000253731.71025.fc

Marci, C. D., & Orr, S. P. (2006). The effect of emotional distance on psychophysiologic concordance and perceived empathy between patient and interviewer. *Applied Psychophysiology Biofeedback, 31*(2), 115–128. https://doi.org/10.1007/s10484-006-9008-4

Maroda, K. J. (2004). *The power of countertransference.* The Analytic Press.

Martín-Brufau, R., Martin-Gorgojo, A., Suso-Ribera, C., Estrada, E., Capriles-Ovalles, M. E., & Romero-Brufau, S. (2020). Emotion regulation strategies, workload conditions, and burnout in healthcare residents. *International Journal of Environmental Research and Public Health, 17*(21), 1–12. https://doi.org/10.3390/ijerph17217816

Martin-Cuellar, A., Lardier, D. T., & Atencio, D. J. (2021). Therapist mindfulness and subjective vitality: The role of psychological wellbeing and compassion satisfaction. *Journal of Mental Health, 30*(1), 113–120. https://doi.org/10.1080/09638237.2019.1644491

Martin, J. S., Goodyear, R. K., & Newton, F. B. (1987). Clinical supervision: An intensive case study. *Professional Psychology: Research and Practice, 18*(3), 225–235. https://doi.org/10.1037/0735-7028.18.3.225

Maslow, A. H. (1943). A theory of human motivation. *Psychological Review, 50*(4), 370–396. https://doi.org/10.1037/h0054346

McCrea, K. T., & Bulanda, J. J. (2008). The practice of compassion in supervision in residential treatment programs for clients with severe mental illness. *Clinical Supervisor, 27*(2), 238–267. https://doi.org/10.1080/07325220802487907

Mehr, K. E., Ladany, N., & Caskie, G. I. L. (2010). Trainee nondisclosure in supervision: What are they not telling you? *Counselling and Psychotherapy Research, 10*(2), 103–113. https://doi.org/10.1080/14733141003712301

Messina, I., Palmieri, A., Sambin, M., Kleinbub, J. R., Voci, A., & Calvo, V. (2013). Somatic underpinnings of perceived empathy: The importance of psychotherapy training. *Psychotherapy Research, 23*(2), 169–177. https://doi.org/10.1080/10503307.2012.748940

Mohammed, W. A., Pappous, A. (Sakis), Muthumayandi, K., & Sharma, D. (2018). The effect of mindfulness meditation on therapists' body-awareness and burnout in different forms of practice. *European Journal of Physiotherapy*, *20*(4), 213–224. https://doi.org/10.1080/21679169.2018.1452980

Mothersole, G. (1999). Parallel process: A review. *Clinical Supervisor*, *18*(2), 107–121. https://doi.org/10.1300/J001v18n02_08

Murison, R. (2016). The neurobiology of stress. In M. Al'Absi & M. A. Flaten (Eds.), *Neuroscience of pain, stress, and emotion: Psychological and clinical implications* (pp. 29–49). Elsevier Inc. https://doi.org/10.1016/b978-0-12-800538-5.00002-9

Neff, K. (2003a). Self-compassion: An alternative conceptualization of a healthy attitude toward oneself self-compassion. *Self and Identity*, *2*, 85–101. https://doi.org/10.1080/15298860390129863

Neff, K. (2003b). The development and validation of a scale to measure self-compassion. *Self and Identity*, *2*, 223–250. https://doi.org/10.1080/15298860390209035

Neff, K. (2011). *Self compassion: Stop beating yourself up and leave insecurity behind*. Hodder & Stoughton.

Neff, K. D., & Germer, C. K. (2013). A pilot study and randomized controlled trial of the mindful self-compassion program. *Journal of Clinical Psychology*, *69*(1), 28–44. https://doi.org/10.1002/jclp.21923

Nelson, J. R., Hall, B. S., Anderson, J. L., Birtles, C., & Hemming, L. (2018). Self–compassion as self-care: A simple and effective tool for counselor educators and counseling students. *Journal of Creativity in Mental Health*, *13*(1), 121–133. https://doi.org/10.1080/15401383.2017.1328292

Nelson, M. L., & Friedlander, M. L. (2001). A close look at conflictual supervisory relationships: The trainee's perspective. *Journal of Counseling Psychology*, *48*(4), 384–395. https://doi.org/10.1037/0022-0167.48.4.384

Newsome, S., Waldo, M., & Gruszka, C. (2012). Mindfulness group work: Preventing stress and increasing self-compassion among helping professionals in training. *Journal for Specialists in Group Work*, *37*(4), 297–311. https://doi.org/10.1080/01933922.2012.690832

Ogden, P. (2018). Polyvagal theory and sensorimotor psychotherapy. In S. W. Porges & D. Dana (Eds.), *Clinical applications of the polyvagal theory: The emergence of polyvagal-informed therapies* (pp. 34–49). W.W. Norton & Company.

Ogden, P., Minton, K., & Pain, C. (2006). *Trauma and the body: A sensorimotor approach to psychotherapy*. W.W. Norton & Company.

Ögren, M. L., Apelman, A., & Klawitter, M. (2002). The group in psychotherapy supervision. *Clinical Supervisor*, *20*(2), 147–175. https://doi.org/10.1300/J001v20n02_12

Päivinen, H., Holma, J., Karvonen, A., Kykyri, V. L., Tsatsishvili, V., Kaartinen, J., Penttonen, M., & Seikkula, J. (2016). Affective arousal during blaming in couple therapy: Combining analyses of verbal discourse and physiological responses in two case studies. *Contemporary Family Therapy*, *38*(4), 373–384. https://doi.org/10.1007/s10591-016-9393-7

Palmieri, A., Kleinbub, J. R., Calvo, V., Benelli, E., Messina, I., Sambin, M., & Voci, A. (2018). Attachment-security prime effect on skin-conductance synchronization in psychotherapists: An empirical study. *Journal of Counseling Psychology*, *65*(4), 490–499. https://doi.org/10.1037/cou0000273

Palmieri, A., Pick, E., Grossman-Giron, A., & Tzur Bitan, D. (2021). Oxytocin as the neurobiological basis of synchronization: A research proposal in psychotherapy settings. *Frontiers in Psychology*, *12*, 1–5. https://doi.org/10.3389/fpsyg.2021.628011

Palumbo, R. V., Marraccini, M. E., Weyandt, L. L., Wilder-Smith, O., McGee, H. A., Liu, S., & Goodwin, M. S. (2017). Interpersonal autonomic physiology: A systematic review of the literature. *Personality and Social Psychology Review*, *21*(2), 99–141. https://doi.org/10.1177/1088868316628405

Park, E. H., Ha, G., Lee, S., Lee, Y. Y., & Lee, S. M. (2019). Relationship between the supervisory working alliance and outcomes: A meta-analysis. *Journal of Counseling and Development*, *97*(4), 437–446. https://doi.org/10.1002/jcad.12292

Porges, S. W. (2011). *The polyvagal theory: Neurophysiological foundations of emotions, attachment, communication and self-regulation*. W.W. Norton & Company.

Porges, S. W. (2017). *The pocket guide to the polyvagal theory: The transformative power of feeling safe*. W.W. Norton & Company.

Pourová, M., Řiháček, T., & Žvelc, G. (2020). Validation of the Czech version of the relational needs satisfaction scale. *Frontiers in Psychology*, *11*, 1–11. https://doi.org/10.3389/fpsyg.2020.00359

Prenn, N. C. N., & Fosha, D. (2017). *Supervision essentials for accelerated experiential dynamic psychotherapy*. American Psychological Association.

Price, C. J., & Hooven, C. (2018). Interoceptive awareness skills for emotion regulation: Theory and approach of mindful awareness in body-oriented therapy (MABT). *Frontiers in Psychology*, *9*, 1–12. https://doi.org/10.3389/fpsyg.2018.00798

Prochazkova, E., & Kret, M. E. (2017). Connecting minds and sharing emotions through mimicry: A neurocognitive model of emotional contagion. *Neuroscience and Biobehavioral Reviews*, *80*, 99–114. https://doi.org/10.1016/j.neubiorev.2017.05.013

Quarto, C. J. (2003). Supervisors' and supervisees' perceptions of control and conflict in counseling supervision. *Clinical Supervisor*, *21*(2), 21–37. https://doi.org/10.1300/J001v21n02_02

Rabinowitz, F. E., Heppner, P. P., & Roehlke, H. J. (1986). Descriptive study of process and outcome variables of supervision over time. *Journal of Counseling Psychology*, *33*(3), 292–300. https://doi.org/10.1037/0022-0167.33.3.292

Racker, H. (1968). *Transference and countertransference*. Karnac.

Ramos-Sánchez, L., Esnil, E., Goodwin, A., Riggs, S., Wright, L. K., Touster, L. O., Ratanasiripong, P., & Rodolfa, E. (2002). Negative supervisory events: Effects on supervision satisfaction and supervisory alliance. *Professional Psychology: Research and Practice*, *33*(2), 197–202. https://doi.org/10.1037/0735-7028.33.2.197

Renfro-Michel, E. L., & Sheperis, C. J. (2009). The relationship between counseling supervisee attachment orientation and perceived bond with supervisor. *Clinical Supervisor*, *28*(2), 141–154. https://doi.org/10.1080/07325220903324306

Richardson, C. M. E., Trusty, W. T., & George, K. A. (2020). Trainee wellness: Self-critical perfectionism, self-compassion, depression, and burnout among doctoral trainees in psychology. *Counselling Psychology Quarterly*, *33*(2), 187–198. https://doi.org/10.1080/09515070.2018.1509839

Riggs, S. A., & Bretz, K. M. (2006). Attachment processes in the supervisory relationship: An exploratory investigation. *Professional Psychology: Research and Practice*, *37*(5), 558–566. https://doi.org/10.1037/0735-7028.37.5.558

Robinson, J. W., Herman, A., & Kaplan, B. J. (1982). Autonomic responses correlate with counselor-client empathy. *Journal of Counseling Psychology*, *29*(2), 195–198. https://doi.org/10.1037/0022-0167.29.2.195

Rockliff, H., Gilbert, P., McEwan, K., Lightman, S., & Glover, D. (2008). A pilot exploration of heart rate variability and salivary cortisol responses to compassion-focused imagery. *Clinical Neuropsychiatry: Journal of Treatment Evaluation, 5*(3), 132–139.

Rothschild, B. (2000). *The body remembers: The psychophysiology of trauma and trauma treatment.* W.W. Norton & Company.

Rothschild, B. (2006). *Help for the helper: The psychophysiology of compassion fatigue and vicarious trauma.* W.W. Norton & Company.

Rothschild, B. (2017). *Body remembers: Revolutionizing trauma treatment* (Vol. 2). W.W. Norton & Company.

Rousmaniere, T. (2017). *Deliberate practice for psychotherapists: A guide to improving clinical effectiveness.* Routledge.

Rožič, T. (2018). Affect regulation in psychotherapy supervision: A multiple case study of moments of change. *Ljetopis Socijalnog Rada [Annual of Social Work], 25*(3), 403–425. https://doi.org/10.3935/ljsr.v25i3.245

Safran, J. D. (2003). The relational turn, the therapeutic alliance, and psychotherapy research: Strange bedfellows or postmodern marriage? *Contemporary Psychoanalysis, 39*(3), 449–475. https://doi.org/10.1080/00107530.2003.10747215

Safran, J. D., & Muran, J. C. (1996). The resolution of ruptures in the therapeutic alliance. *Journal of Consulting and Clinical Psychology, 64*(3), 447–458. https://doi.org/10.1037/0022-006X.64.3.447

Safran, J. D., & Muran, J. C. (2000). *Negotiating the therapeutic alliance: A relational treatment guide.* Guilford Press.

Safran, J. D., Muran, J. C., Stevens, C., & Rothman, M. (2008). A relational approach to supervision: Addressing ruptures in the alliance. In C. A. Falender & E. P. Shafranske (Eds.), *Casebook for clinical supervision: A competency-based approach* (pp. 137–157). American Psychological Association. https://doi.org/10.1037/11792-007

Saxbe, D., & Repetti, R. L. (2010). For better or worse? Coregulation of couples' cortisol levels and mood states. *Journal of Personality and Social Psychology, 98*(1), 92–103. https://doi.org/10.1037/a0016959

Saxbe, D. E., Margolin, G., Spies Shapiro, L., Ramos, M., Rodriguez, A., & Iturralde, E. (2014). Relative influences: Patterns of HPA axis concordance during triadic family interaction. *Health Psychology, 33*(3), 273–281. https://doi.org/10.1037/a0033509

Sayers, W. M., Creswell, J. D., & Taren, A. (2015). The emerging neurobiology of mindfulness and emotion processing. In B. D. Ostafin, M. D. Robinson, & B. P. Meier (Eds.), *Handbook of mindfulness and self-regulation* (pp. 9–22). Springer. https://doi.org/10.1007/978-1-4939-2263-5_2

Schore, A. N. (1994). *Affect regulation and the origin of the self.* Lawrence Erlbaum Associates.

Schore, A. N. (2019). *Right brain psychotherapy.* W.W. Norton & Company.

Scoglio, A. A. J., Rudat, D. A., Garvert, D., Jarmolowski, M., Jackson, C., & Herman, J. L. (2015). Self-compassion and responses to trauma: The role of emotion regulation. *Journal of Interpersonal Violence, 33*(3), 2016–2036. https://doi.org/10.1177/0886260515622296

Searles, H. F. (1955). The informational value of the supervisor's emotional experiences. *Psychiatry, 18*(2), 135–146. https://doi.org/10.1080/00332747.1955.11023001

Sedighimornani, N., Rimes, K. A., & Verplanken, B. (2019). Exploring the relationships between mindfulness, self-compassion, and shame. *SAGE Open, 9*(3). 215824401986629. https://doi.org/10.1177/2158244019866294

Senior, M., & Shotter, A. (2007, April 12–15). *The difficult to love client* [Workshop]. International Integrative Psychotherapy Association Conference, Rome, Italy.

Seth, A. K. (2013). Interoceptive inference, emotion, and the embodied self. *Trends in Cognitive Sciences, 17*(11), 565–573. https://doi.org/10.1016/j.tics.2013.09.007

Shapiro, S. L., Brown, K. W., & Biegel, G. M. (2007). Teaching self-care to caregivers: Effects of mindfulness-based stress reduction on the mental health of therapists in training. *Training and Education in Professional Psychology, 1*(2), 105–115. https://doi.org/10.1037/1931-3918.1.2.105

Siegel, D. J. (1999). *The developing mind: Toward a neurobiology of interpersonal experience.* The Guilford Press.

Siegel, D. J. (2007). *The mindful brain: Reflection and attunement in the cultivation of well being.* W.W. Norton & Company.

Siegel, D. J. (2012). *The developing mind: How relationships and the brain interact to shape who we are* (2nd ed.). The Guilford Press.

Siegel, R. D., & Germer, C. K. (2012). Wisdom and compassion: Two wings of a bird. In C. K. Germer & D. J. Siegel (Eds.), *Wisdom and compassion in psychotherapy: Deepening mindfulness in clinical practice* (pp. 7–34). The Guilford Press.

Singer, T., & Klimecki, O. M. (2014). Empathy and compassion. *Current Biology, 24*(18), R875–R878. https://doi.org/10.1016/j.cub.2014.06.054

Stewart, L. (2010). Relational needs of the therapist: Countertransference, clinical work and supervision. Benefits and disruptions in psychotherapy. *International Journal of Integrative Psychotherapy, 1*(1), 41–50.

Stolorow, R. D. (1994). The intersubjective context of intrapsychic experience. In R. D. Stolorow, G. E. Atwood, & B. Brandschaft (Eds.), *The intersubjective perspective* (pp. 3–15). Jason Aronson.

Stoltenberg, C. D., & McNeill, B. W. (2009). *IDM supervision: An integrative developmental model for supervising counselors and therapists.* Routledge.

Strozier, A. L., Barnett-Queen, T., & Bennett, C. K. (2000). Supervision: Critical process and outcome variables. *Clinical Supervisor, 19*(1), 21–39. https://doi.org/10.1300/J001v19n01_02

Suveg, C., Shaffer, A., & Davis, M. (2016). Family stress moderates relations between physiological and behavioral synchrony and child self-regulation in mother-preschooler dyads. *Developmental Psychobiology, 58*(1), 83–97. https://doi.org/10.1002/dev.21358

Talbot, N. L. (1995). Unearthing shame in the supervisory relationship. *American Journal of Psychotherapy, 49*(3), 338–349.

Taren, A. A., Creswell, J. D., & Gianaros, P. J. (2013). Dispositional mindfulness covaries with smaller amygdala and caudate volumes in community adults. *PLoS ONE, 8*(5), 1–7. https://doi.org/10.1371/journal.pone.0064574

Taylor, J. H., Poole, S., Rodway, R., & Tyson, R. (2006). Parallel process in supervision: A qualitative investigation. *Europen Journal of Qualitative Research in Psychotherapy, 1*, 10–20.

Teper, R., & Inzlicht, M. (2013). Meditation, mindfulness and executive control: The importance of emotional acceptance and brain-based performance monitoring.

Social Cognitive and Affective Neuroscience, 8(1), 85–92. https://doi.org/10.1093/scan/nss045

Teper, R., Segal, Z. V., & Inzlicht, M. (2013). Inside the mindful mind: How mindfulness enhances emotion regulation through improvements in executive control. *Current Directions in Psychological Science, 22*(6), 449–454. https://doi.org/10.1177/0963721413495869

Thomas, J. T. (2007). Informed consent through contracting for supervision: Minimizing risks, enhancing benefits. *Professional Psychology: Research and Practice, 38*, 221–231. https://doi.org/10.1037/0735-7028.38.3.221

Toksoy, Ş., Cerit, C., Aker, A., & Žvelc, G. (2020). Relational needs satisfaction scale: Reliability and validity study in Turkish. *Anatolian Journal of Psychiatry, 21*(0), 37–44. https://doi.org/10.5455/apd.115143

Tracey, T. J. G., Bludworth, J., & Glidden-Tracey, C. E. (2012). Are there parallel processes in psychotherapy supervision? An empirical examination. *Psychotherapy, 49*(3), 330–343. https://doi.org/10.1037/a0026246

Tschacher, W., & Meier, D. (2019). Physiological synchrony in psychotherapy sessions. *Psychotherapy Research*, 1–16. https://doi.org/10.1080/10503307.2019.1612114

Uršič, N., & Žvelc, G. (2017, September 20–22). Compassion in psychotherapy: Views and experiences of psychotherapists [Conference presentation]. *Society for Psychotherapy Research UK & European Chapters, 4th Joint Conference.*

Uvnäs-Moberg, K., Handlin, L., & Petersson, M. (2014). Self-soothing behaviors with particular reference to oxytocin release induced by non-noxious sensory stimulation. *Frontiers in Psychology, 5*, 1–16. https://doi.org/10.3389/fpsyg.2014.01529

Vago, D. R., & Silbersweig, D. A. (2012). Self-awareness, self-regulation, and self-transcendence (S-ART): A framework for understanding the neurobiological mechanisms of mindfulness. *Frontiers in Human Neuroscience, 6*, 1–30. https://doi.org/10.3389/fnhum.2012.00296

van der Brink, E., & Koster, F. (2015). *Mindfulness-based compassionate living.* Routledge.

Vettese, L. C., Dyer, C. E., Li, W. L., & Wekerle, C. (2011). Does self-compassion mitigate the association between childhood maltreatment and later emotion regulation difficulties? A preliminary investigation. *International Journal of Mental Health and Addiction, 9*(5), 480–491. https://doi.org/10.1007/s11469-011-9340-7

Vîşcu, L.-I., & Watkins, E. C. (2021). *A guide to clinical supervision: The supervision pyramid.* Elsevier.

Voon, S. P., Lau, P. L., Leong, K. E., & Jaafar, J. L. S. (2021). Self-compassion and psychological well-being among Malaysian counselors: The mediating role of resilience. *Asia-Pacific Education Researcher, 31*, 475–488. https://doi.org/10.1007/s40299-021-00590-w

Watkins, C. E. (1995). Pathological attachment styles in psychotherapy supervision. *Psychotherapy, 32*(2), 333–340. https://doi.org/10.1037/0033-3204.32.2.333

Watkins, C. E. (2012). Some thoughts about parallel process and psychotherapy supervision: When is a parallel just a parallel? *Psychotherapy, 49*(3), 344–346. https://doi.org/10.1037/a0029191

Watkins, C. E. (2014). The supervisory alliance: A half century of theory, practice, and research in critical perspective. *American Journal of Psychotherapy, 68*(1), 19–55. https://doi.org/10.1176/appi.psychotherapy.2014.68.1.19

Watkins, C. E. (2017a). Convergence in psychotherapy supervision: A common factors, common processes, common practices perspective. *Journal of Psychotherapy Integration*, *27*(2), 140–152. https://doi.org/10.1037/int0000040

Watkins, C. E. (2017b). How does psychotherapy supervision work? Contributions of connection, conception, allegiance, alignment, and action. *Journal of Psychotherapy Integration*, *27*(2), 201–217. https://doi.org/10.1037/int0000058

Watkins, C. E. (2018a). The supervisee's internal supervisor representations: Their role in stimulating psychotherapist development. *International Journal of Psychotherapy*, *22*(3), 63–73.

Watkins, C. E. (2018b). The supervision pyramid: A commonalities-based synthesis of intervention, relationship, and person/personhood. *American Journal of Psychotherapy*, *71*(3), 88–94. https://doi.org/10.1176/appi.psychotherapy.20180017

Watkins, C. E. (2021). Rupture and rupture repair in clinical supervision: Some thoughts and steps along the way. *Clinical Supervisor*, *40*(2), 321–344. https://doi.org/10.1080/07325223.2021.1890657

Watkins, C. E., Hook, J. N., Mosher, D. K., & Callahan, J. L. (2019). Humility in clinical supervision: Fundamental, foundational, and transformational. *Clinical Supervisor*, *38*(1), 58–78. https://doi.org/10.1080/07325223.2018.1487355

Watkins, C. E., Reyna, S. H., Ramos, M. J., & Hook, J. N. (2015). The ruptured supervisory alliance and its repair: On supervisor apology as a reparative intervention. *Clinical Supervisor*, *34*(1), 98–114. https://doi.org/10.1080/07325223.2015.1015194

Watkins, C. E. , Vîşcu, L.-I., Cădariu, I.-E., & Žvelc, M. (2021). Problematic self-efficacy inferences in beginning psychotherapy supervisees: Identification and management. *Journal of Contemporary Psychotherapy*, *52*, 109–116. https://doi.org/10.1007/s10879-021-09525-4

White, V. E., & Queener, J. (2003). Supervisor and supervisee attachments and social provisions related to the supervisory working alliance. *Counselor Education and Supervision*, *42*(3), 203–218. https://doi.org/10.1002/j.1556-6978.2003.tb01812.x

Worthen, V., & McNeill, B. W. (1996). A phenomenological investigation of "good" supervision events. *Journal of Counseling Psychology*, *43*(1), 25–34. https://doi.org/10.1037/0022-0167.43.1.25

Worthington, E. L. (2006). Changes in supervision as counselors and supervisors gain experience: A review. *Training and Education in Professional Psychology*, *S*(2), 133–160. https://doi.org/10.1037/1931-3918.s.2.133

Worthington, E. L., & Roehlke, H. J. (1979). Effective supervision as perceived by beginning counselors-in-training. *Journal of Counseling Psychology*, *26*(1), 64–73. https://doi.org/10.1037/0022-0167.26.1.64

Yaribeygi, H., Panahi, Y., Sahraei, H., Johnston, T. P., & Sahebkar, A. (2017). The impact of stress on body function: A review. *EXCLI Journal*, *16*, 1057–1072. https://doi.org/10.17179/excli2017-480

Yip, S. Y. C., Mak, W. W. S., Chio, F. H. N., & Law, R. W. (2017). The mediating role of self-compassion between mindfulness and compassion fatigue among therapists in Hong Kong. *Mindfulness*, *8*(2), 460–470. https://doi.org/10.1007/s12671-016-0618-5

Žvelc, G. (2009). Between self and others: Relational schemas as an integrating construct in psychotherapy. *Transactional Analysis Journal*, *39*(1), 22–38. https://doi.org/10.1177/036215370903900104

Žvelc, G. (2010). Relational schemas theory and transactional analysis. *Transactional Analysis Journal, 40*(1), 8–22. https://doi.org/10.1177/036215371004000103

Žvelc, G. (2012). Mindful processing in psychotherapy: Facilitating natural healing process within attuned therapeutic relationship. *International Journal of Integrative Psychotherapy, 3*(1), 42–58.

Žvelc, G. (2014). Two aware minds are more powerful than only one: Mindfulness, relational schemas, and integrating adult. In K. Tudor & G. Summers (Eds.), *Co-creative transactional analysis: Papers, responses, dialogues, and developments* (pp. 165–170). Karnac Books.

Žvelc, G., Jovanoska, K., & Žvelc, M. (2020). Development and validation of the relational needs satisfaction scale. *Frontiers in Psychology, 11*, 1–15. https://doi.org/10.3389/fpsyg.2020.00901

Žvelc, G., & Žvelc, M. (2008, July 1–4). The power of present moment: Mindful processing in psychotherapy and counseling [Conference session]. *Conference on Positive Psychology*, Opatija, Croatia.

Žvelc, G., & Žvelc, M. (2009, April 17–19). Loss and regain of 'now': Transforming trauma through mindful processing [Conference session]. *4th International Integrative Psychotherapy Conference*, Bled, Slovenia.

Žvelc, G., & Žvelc, M. (2021). *Integrative psychotherapy: A mindfulness- and compassion-oriented approach.* Routledge.

Žvelc, M. (2008). Working with mistakes in psychotherapy: A relational model. *European Journal for Qualitative Research in Psychotherapy, 3*, 1–9.

Žvelc, M. (2013). Defining psychotherapy supervision and understanding supervisor functioning. In A. Podlesek (Ed.), *The development of the supervised practice of psychologists in Slovenia* (pp. 39–50). University Press, Faculty of Arts.

Žvelc, M. (2015). Pomembni dogodki v superviziji: Izkušnje in pogledi supervizantov [Significant events in psychotherapy supervision: Supervisees' experiences and perspectives]. *KAIROS—Slovenian Journal of Psychotherapy, 9*(1–2), 51–81.

Žvelc, M. (2017). *Razvoj modela spodbujajočih in ovirajočih dejavnikov v superviziji psihoterapije [Neobjavljena doktorska disertacija] [Development of a model of facilitating and hindering factors in psychotherapy supervision. Unpublished doctoral dissertation].* Univerza v Ljubljani.

Žvelc, M., & Žvelc, G. (2021). Supervisees' experience of non-disclosure in psychotherapy supervision. *Ljetopis Socijalnog Rada [Annual of Social Work], 28*(1), 231–256. https://doi.org/10.3935/ljsr.v28i1.330

Index